UNLOCK YOUR POWER, REMEMBER
YOUR MAGIC, LOVE YOUR BODY

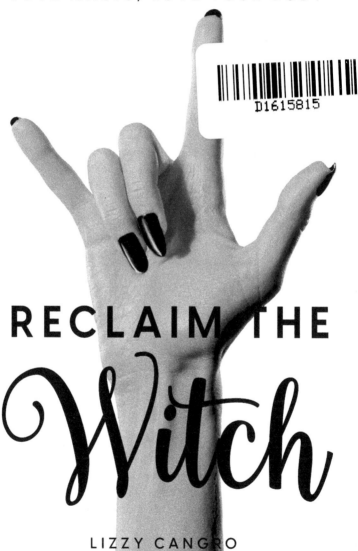

D1615815

RECLAIM THE

Witch

LIZZY CANGRO

To download your free companion journal pages, go to
www.reclaimthewitch.com

Ordering information: special discounts are available on quantity purchases by corporations, associations, and others. For details, contact
lizzy@nutritionbylizzy.com

Medical Disclaimer:
The information contained in this book is intended for educational and informational purposes only. It is not intended to be a substitute for professional medical advice, diagnosis, or treatment. Always seek the advice of a qualified healthcare provider with any questions you may have regarding a medical condition.

Privacy notice:
The names and identifying details of individuals mentioned in this work have been changed to protect their privacy. The events and experiences described in this work are based on true accounts, but some of the names and identifying details have been altered to ensure the anonymity of those involved.

To woman power...

Contents

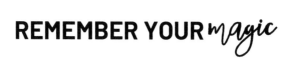

REMEMBER YOUR *magic*

Close your eyes, take a deep breath, and remember that feeling you once had as a child. That incredible sense of freedom where you embraced the magic of life, believed anything was possible, and felt at peace within your body.

Before you were told and sold impossible standards for how to look, eat, and move.

Before you were taught to hide your power and play small.

Before you questioned your worth and felt you needed others' permission and approval to be yourself.

I remember this feeling as vividly as the day it was taken from me.

I was seven years old and on a day trip to the beach with my mum's parents. When grandad parked next to my favorite wooden playground, I knew it was going to be a good day.

After hours of playing in the arcade and being refreshed by the salty sea air whipping against my rosy cheeks as we walked along the promenade, I was bouncing with excitement to run around the playground before we went home.

As I let go of my nan's hand and skipped towards the wooden frame, I could see another girl my age playing in the sand. Forgetting my shyness, I boldly went over and introduced myself. "Hi, my name is Lizzy, and…I'm a witch."

She abruptly stopped making patterns in the sand with her finger, gave me one glance, and fled across the playground to her mother in horrified silence.

Feelings of confusion and powerlessness filled my tiny body as I traipsed back over to my nan, and we walked back to my grandad and the car. I didn't fully understand what had happened, and I needed comfort and reassurance from someone.

"What did I do?" I asked my nan.

On the drive home, she told my grandad that I had just told another little girl that I was a witch, which caused the entire car to erupt in laughter.

I sank into my seat and half laughed along. Of course, I wasn't a witch! How crazy of me to think so, right?

Wrong.

Little Lizzy should have celebrated in that moment. It was the day that I spoke the powerful truth: that I was magic and that we are all magic. Instead of being encouraged, I was mocked.

From a primitive survival standpoint, my subconscious knew it wasn't safe for this to happen. Being viewed as crazy by your family and being kicked out of your "tribe" is the last thing a dependent child wants. So, instead of stepping any further into my power, I ran from it.

It wasn't until several decades later, as I was listening to a podcast with a medicine woman called "Sand," that I found the comfort and validation I needed to reawaken my inner witch and begin my journey of healing the years I spent in self-suppression.

On the podcast, Sand shared her own story of hiding her magic after being publicly shamed and blamed for being able to "see" a family friend's deceased son when she was a little girl. As an adult, she started to get nightly visits from ancestors, encouraging her to remember her magic. Sand's story was so relatable and reassured me that I wasn't alone.

You, sister, are not alone. Millions of women just like you are ready to let go of the narrative that makes us feel as if we're "not good enough," lacking in something, and we should be ashamed of who we are. These women are ready to confidently step into the body they love, create trusting relationships with other women, and unite on the journey of rediscovering the witch within. The fact that you're here reading this tells me you want this, too.

However, if you're like me, it may feel overwhelming, and you may not know where to start. *Reclaim the Witch* is designed to be a step-by-step beginner's guide for women that takes you by the hand and lovingly walks you through the amazing (and sometimes scary) journey of unlocking your power, embracing your magic, and loving your body.

I'll be revealing *The Curse, The Cure, The Witchual* and *The Wisdom* of 11 important steps on your journey. *The Curse* is a problem that you will encounter, *The Cure* is my remedy for this problem, and *The Witchual* is a tool, or collection of tools that you can use to achieve *The Cure*. Meanwhile, *The Wisdom* provides a summary of each step.

The tools I share are for educational purposes only and aren't a substitute for professional support and advice. I'm not here to tell you what to do (because, let's face it, who wants *another* self-help book?) and, just like I wouldn't prescribe you a cookie-cutter meal plan, I'm not going to prescribe you a rigid routine. Instead, it's my intention to provide you with some tools for you to play with so that you can reactivate your magic in a way that feels good to *you*.

While I share my favorite tools, I acknowledge that they aren't the only witchy tools out there. I was selective in the tools I included and divided the book into manageable sections to make the book easier to digest and encourage you to act from a position of empowerment.

An empowered woman who believes in herself and rebels against the status quo is dangerous for a structure that is often referred to as "the patriarchy." For the purposes of this book, I will define the patriarchy as a system dominated by wounded masculine energy. It is not a person, and it is not a gender. It is an agenda. The agenda is to keep us all in line. In doing so, it makes money from our insecurities (just look at the diet industry), takes away our freedom (see the train wreck of a case with *Roe v. Wade*), and sucks our souls dry (hello, corporate America).

But what if it didn't have to be this way?

What if you remembered your magic?

What if you remembered you *are* magic?

Warning! This process of remembering will require you to "get messy." At times, you will need to be vulnerable and clear out old beliefs that are no longer serving you. You might also feel yourself yo-yoing between sadness, anger, anxiety, and excitement along the way; these and every other emotion you feel are valid and contain pearls of wisdom if you allow yourself to go there.

And I really do hope you go there. Because not only will allowing yourself to get messy benefit you, but you are also paving a realistic and attainable way for other women to step out of their comfort zones and into their power zones, if they so choose. After all, the point of reclaiming our power is not to dominate but to give people the freedom to choose, right?

Some women may not be ready, but when we *do* choose to reclaim our power? Woah! Get ready for some very cool, magical stuff.

Are *you* ready, sister?

STEP 1: *Wake* UP

The Curse

For two years, I was being hunted by an evil witch who visited my parents' house. She would ask for me whenever my mum answered the door. I was so frightened the witch would find me that I would hide behind the sofa in the living room until she left. As I huddled behind the sofa, I prayed that she would go away and never come back. But she always did.

If you're like me, you've probably had a few scary dreams over the years. This recurring dream terrified me.

Until I began to learn how to interpret dreams (spoiler alert: I'll be teaching you how to do this later), I didn't realize it was a sign that, even as a tiny human, I was aware of my magic…and feared it. Somehow, I knew I was powerful, but the patriarchy had already planted the seed in my mind that this also meant I was evil.

At the tender ages of eight and nine years old, was I *really* an evil person? Of course not. But this was already embedded in my subconscious and impacting not only my dreams but also my thoughts, feelings, and behaviors in my waking life. For example, I felt guilty every time I set boundaries with other people or expressed my needs. I would label it "selfish" and put myself last to try to please others and prove I was a "good" person. It was the opposite of being in my power.

Maybe you can relate to some of these thoughts, feelings, and behaviors?

Maybe you see them in your mother?

Your grandmother?

Your daughter?

Your friends?

It chills me to think how many other women are having their magic dialed down or, worse, extinguished by the subliminal patriarchal messages about being powerful, what it means to be a "good" (enough) person, and the impact this is ultimately having on their lives. From my 12-year-old cousin who self-harms to my friend's 10-year-old who thinks she's "fat," it's especially heartbreaking for me to see how these messages are hurting women at such an early age.

It also lights a big fire within my belly to want to tip the balance back in favor of the witch—the woman who stands in her power and owns her magic. The good news is that every one of us can do this for ourselves. The bad news is that pointing our wands and playing the victim isn't going to help.

Instead, we need to be responsible for reclaiming our power by taking an honest look at our subconscious stories. The easiest way to access these is through our dreams, when our conscious brain is at rest.

When I first started choosing to reclaim my power and own my magic, my dreams became very potent. I had one dream where I was in the middle of a large forest fire with a group of old classmates who were all trying to escape. Out of nowhere, I heard a woman's voice say, "Always go back to the elder tree." I then saw a silhouetted, large, ancient elder tree that was safe from the fire. I woke up knowing that the message and imagery were significant, but I had no idea what an elder tree symbolized. So, like any millennial, I Googled it:

The tree was sacred across Northern Europe, and the Druids regarded it as a gift from the Earth Mother who lived within it…The plant's ability to sprout from damaged boughs…symbolized regeneration.[1]

This was as far as my dream interpretation went, and, for about six months, I continued having vivid dreams without understanding what my subconscious was trying to tell me. That all changed on the night of a partial lunar eclipse, which was the longest of its kind in 580 years.[2]

As women, the moon can have a significant impact on our mood and energy levels (more on this in Step 4: Get PsCyclic), and all day I was tired, emotional, and a little reactive. No matter how hard I tried to fight it, this only ramped up and up as the peak of the eclipse approached. I felt like I'd drank ten glasses of wine as I watched the beautiful red moon disappear and reappear. By the time it had finished, I was so lethargic that I could barely lift my head. With the help of my husband, I hauled myself over to bed and crashed immediately.

That night, I dreamt of the shaman I wanted to work with. Shamans are healers who use altered states of consciousness to communicate with the spirit realm. I hadn't seen a picture of what this shaman looked like, but I just knew it was him in my dream. He asked me whether I had been vaccinated against COVID-19, and, when I said "yes," he told me to go upstairs to a waiting room with hundreds of other people who also wanted to work with him.

Being the impatient person that I am, I couldn't bear waiting. So, in my stubbornness, I left the room and decided to make my own journey "home," where I kept encountering these huge physical barriers. First, there was a big gate completely blocking the entrance to the subway. Next, an insurmountable wall. The imagery was so rich that, when I woke up, I knew this meant something significant and I needed to decipher it. But how?

The Cure

Have you ever had the sense that your dream was telling you something? Rather than disregarding this as "woo woo" and weird, I encourage you to get curious about what your subconscious is trying to communicate via the messages and stories encoded in your dreams.

I first became aware of the potential my dreams held while my husband and I were vacationing in Las Vegas and staying at the New York, New York Hotel. I had begun to frequently dream about witches. One dream that particularly stood out to me was about a coven that I belonged to, where the high priestess gave me and another witch a task to complete. The dream ended with the high priestess pushing us off the top of the New York, New York roller coaster as a punishment because we botched the assignment we were given.

How clever is it that our subconscious pulls metaphors from our waking lives to communicate with us?! When we dig into these metaphors a little more in a minute, you'll see that this dream was about me learning to use my magic but being afraid of messing up and making mistakes. I was aware that there were others who were further along on their journey, and I feared that they would judge me or kick me out of their group. I was also aware that there were others like me who were learning and that, as humans, we all make mistakes, especially as we're learning.

Decoding my dreams has been a total game changer because it's helped me reveal my hidden internal narratives – and shift them when needed. I'll be discussing the importance of our stories more in Step 5: Spell it Out. For now, I highly encourage you to learn how to interpret your dreams. The more you do this, the more you'll connect with your subconscious. The more you connect to your subconscious and the stories stored within it, the more you'll step into your power because, incredibly, 95% of your brain's power is held in the subconscious.[3]

The Witchual

Remember Your Dreams

A pre-requisite for dream interpretation is that you *actually* remember your dreams! I know; easier said than done. That's where keeping a dream journal comes in handy. This is a notebook you keep by the side of your bed to note down any imagery, messages, or feelings you receive in your dreams each night.

Here's an example taken from my dream journal:

> January 24th, 2023: Slept heavy with dream re: our wedding. I felt like I didn't fit in among groups of people at the wedding + just wanted to rebel. So, I went off the beaten path and jumped in a cold-water stream with a couple of our closest friends. After that we went and bought lots of copies of my book from independent bookstores which messed up the sales for a large national bookstore.
>
> January 25th, 2023: Dreamt about gang shooting, Mum/Dad/me had to quickly leave our home because of the imminent danger.

Logging your dreams will take you less than five minutes every morning, and having a fancy notebook isn't necessary. For your convenience, I've included journal pages at the back of this book for you to use. Alternatively, some people prefer to use a voice recorder to document their dreams.

Whether you use a physical or audio dream journal, it's important to log as much detail as you can right after you wake up. That's because our dreams are held in a part of our brain that only deals with short-term memory. Just think about any time you've tried to recount a dream to somebody later in the day only to realize you've forgotten it; that dream was not stored in your long-term memory, so remembering it at that point becomes impossible. Unless, of course, you have a dream journal.

Look for Associations

Once you have a dream recorded, you can start to decode it. The most effective way to do this is to consider your associations with the imagery, people, words, and sensations from the dream. For example, I associate witches with women in their power, magic, and the occult. I associate rollercoasters with fun, fear, difficulties, and life's journey. As the saying goes, "Life is a rollercoaster."

Please refrain from using a dream dictionary when decoding your dreams. Dream dictionaries are so prescriptive and don't account for your own interpretations of what certain things mean. With dream dictionaries, rather than listening to yourself, you end up listening to whoever wrote the dictionary and relying on *their* interpretations, which may be different from yours. For example, you have a dream of a snake, and the dream dictionary tells you a snake represents transformation. However, you're scared of snakes so what the snake really represents for you is fear. See the difference?

Take Conscious Action

After you've deciphered the metaphors in your dream, take a conscious action that symbolizes to your subconscious that you've received and understood the message it was trying to communicate. Going back to my earlier dream about witches in Vegas as an example, I could have taken the conscious action of going on the rollercoaster to show my subconscious that, while I was scared on this journey, I was safe and not alone. Instead, I shared the dream with my mentor, who was teaching me about dream interpretation. This discussion reinforced to my subconscious that the "high priestess" was supporting me, and I didn't need to worry about "getting it wrong."

Side note: I highly recommend having the support of an expert on your journey to waking up to your power, you can also enlist the support of the universe. You can do this several ways, including by asking for support in your head as you meditate or by speaking your request out loud.

I asked for guidance following the dream I had on the night of the eclipse by saying in my head, "Please guide me, Universe." Yep, it's that simple. The following day, I found a black onyx pendant at a local street market. It had a tree of life wired around it, and I knew instantly that it was my sign from the universe that I had asked for. Later, I looked up what black onyx represents: grounding and protection against negative energy.[4] The tree of life, on the other hand, represents personal growth and rebirth.[5]

I carried the pendant in my wallet wherever I went as a reminder of how the universe had my back during this time of huge personal growth. I always felt safe and at peace whenever I saw it among my quarters. It suddenly disappeared about a month later. My subconscious knew I had received the message and I no longer needed the pendant, so the universe sent the pendant on its way to help someone else. And that's the amazing thing: When our subconscious and the universe collaborate, switching on our powers becomes that much easier.

The Wisdom

The irony isn't lost on me that, to wake up to our magic and unlock our power, we must first dive deep into our dreams. Our subconscious communicates powerful messages to us when we dream in the form of metaphors, which we can decode and use to inform our waking lives. The simple 3-step witchual above will help you do this for yourself.

I understand that it can be frustrating if you struggle to get enough sleep in the first place. If you're someone who has difficulty sleeping, DM me on Instagram @nutritionbylizzy with the phrase 'sleep help' and one of my expert witches will send over some nutrition and lifestyle tips so that you can improve your sleep and gain better access to the potent power of your dreams tonight.

STEP 2: S-Witch ON YOUR POWERS

The Curse

In the last section, I told you about the time I manifested a black onyx pendant. It may not sound very impressive, but when it happened, I felt like Sabrina the Teenage Witch and was in total awe of my magical powers. I wanted more.

After pondering what I did to cause this seemingly miraculous manifestation, I realized the key was simply having an all-knowing certainty that something good was about to happen and surrendering to the process of that becoming a reality. I then saw how this paralleled all the other wondrous manifestations in my life, including the time I manifested the man I married.

I remember it like it was yesterday. I walked along the Hermosa Beach strand in March 2018, with the warmth of the sun kissing my fair English skin, and suddenly I heard myself think the most random thought with absolute conviction: "I'm going to marry an American one day." Three years later, I married my sexy Southern Californian roommate, Steve.

However, in March 2018, I'd only just met Steve and was dating someone else at the time, so I could never have consciously predicted that he and I would get married. All I had was an intuitive nudge.

I had this same nudge again in December 2020, this time about writing a book that gives women tools to stop dieting, silence their inner mean girl, and confidently step into the body they love. I woke up one morning, turned to Steve, and said, "I think I need to write a book." A year later, I published *Reclaim the Rebel*.

Manifestation has become somewhat of a buzzword thanks to social media, and I love the fact that this publicity has helped people become aware of the fact that they're magic; that they have the power to create their desired reality. However, it's become so commercialized and pushed in our faces that, rather than trusting that 'all-knowing' feeling and sitting back to let things naturally manifest, we force the process.

Maybe you've encountered the gurus trying to sell you their $1000 courses that promise to teach you how to manifest your greatest desires within four weeks. Sounds good, doesn't it?

But that's not how manifestation works. The universe is like Flash, everyone's favorite Zootopia sloth: it doesn't work to your schedule, and it certainly doesn't respond to being cajoled by overachievers and those who have little patience. And yes, I'm totally speaking from personal experience here!

In contrast, whenever I've brought wonderful things into my life, nothing has needed to be forced to make my all-knowing feeling a reality. Yes, I took action. For example, I left an unhealthy relationship and sat down to write my book every day for two months. But it never felt like I was pushing. It was more like a gentle pull; I just sat back, stayed in alignment with what I valued, and from that place I could magnetically attract what I really wanted.

The Cure

Being in alignment is essential for manifestation. The universe is always working in your best interest (even if you don't always feel like it is) and, as a result, won't let you manifest anything that doesn't correspond with your subconscious values. Being clear on what these values are and whether you're in situations that align with them can therefore be super helpful in switching on your manifestation powers.

Start by asking yourself questions like:

▽ Does this feel good to me?
▽ What do I *really* value?
▽ Does this align with what I value?
▽ Do I believe this could happen for me?

Get super honest with yourself, even if the answer feels uncomfortable or unexpected.

Then, take an action that helps you maintain or realign with your values. It doesn't have to be a massive step like moving countries or changing careers. It could be dedicating 15 minutes of your day to write, move your body, or do something you absolutely love.

If you find in answering the above questions that you don't believe that you're capable or worthy of manifesting your deepest desires, go to www.reclaimthewitch.com and book a call with me so we can discuss how you can shift that so that your subconscious stories about your worth and capabilities are aligned with what you consciously want.

Your manifestation powers come from your subconscious working in conjunction with you being in aligned action. To access your subconscious, you need to be in a relaxed state where your brain waves are at a slower frequency than when you are in conscious thought.

When you're in conscious thought, planning "how to" get what you want and trying to make sense of things when they *do* happen, you'll tend to overthink and overanalyze, and in doing so, switch off your magical manifestation abilities.

Contrary to what you may have been led to believe, putting yourself into a state of relaxation does not necessarily mean you need to sit in a dark room and meditate for hours on end in complete stillness and silence. If this makes you feel relaxed; go for it. If, on the other hand, you're like me and this makes you want to pull your hair out, try something else.

Through experimentation, I've found several things that efficiently calm my nervous system and help slow my brain waves; daydreaming while walking in nature, self-hypnosis, and breathwork. Maybe your relaxation portals are similar; maybe they're different. It's not really what you use to relax you but a matter of knowing what works best for you and using it. That's the beauty of reclaiming your power; you have total agency over your choices.

The Witchual

In *Reclaim the Rebel*, I talk about how part of my daily routine includes 15 minutes of self-hypnosis in the morning and in the evening. This is a powerful tool for helping me relax at the start and end of the day, take time for myself, even when I'm busy, and switch on my manifestation powers.

My self-hypnosis audio takes me through a series of deep breaths to calm my nervous system and put me in a more receptive state for manifesting. It then guides me to imagine what it will look like, feel like, and sound like when I achieve my desires.

While audio can be helpful, and I can recommend some very skilled hypnotherapists who you can work with, you can also do this exercise by yourself. Find a nice, quiet, and comfortable spot where you won't be disturbed for 15 minutes. I recommend sitting up as opposed to lying down so that you don't fall asleep (it's not a problem if you do; it just means your body really needed the rest, so honor that, too).

Start by taking some long, slow, deep breaths in through your nose and out through your mouth. I practice box breathing, where you breathe in for the count of four, hold for four, breathe out for four, hold for four. Repeat five to ten times, noticing yourself feeling increasingly relaxed.

Then, start to create a scene in your mind where you're in the future and you have everything you want in life. What do you see? What do you hear? How do you feel? Allow yourself to really sink into the vision. Who are you with? What do you look like? What are you doing?

If you start to notice you're overthinking things—for example, you may be asking, "How do I make this happen?" The remedy is simple: redirect your focus back to a place of relaxation by taking a couple of long, deep breaths.

Spend as much time as you want to enjoy your future playing out as a movie in your mind. When you are ready, count yourself up from one to five, gradually becoming increasingly aware of your body (start to wiggle your toes and figures) and surroundings (gently open your eyes).

Do this first thing in the morning when you wake up and last thing at night before you go to bed. If you stay consistent with this simple practice, you'll very quickly discover things in your life shifting towards what you desire without you having to do anything whatsoever. Within weeks, one of my clients told me how it felt like magic when she stopped mindlessly snacking despite decades of emotional eating. It is magic, and best of all, it's *your* magic!

The Wisdom

We all have the power to manifest what we desire in life, from amazing health to incredible wealth. To effortlessly attract what we desire without force or frustration, it's important that we feel relaxed and totally aligned with what we are asking from the universe. Head on over to www.reclaimthewitch.com and claim the self-hypnosis audio I use every day so that you can easily put yourself into this state.

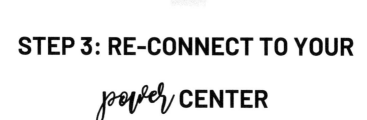

STEP 3: RE-CONNECT TO YOUR

power CENTER

The Curse

I feel like we have gotten to know one another a bit better now that I've assisted you in waking up and switching on your powers. So, I'll let you in on a little something about me: two of my favorite topics are health and wellness.

Okay, so maybe this isn't such a big secret, considering I'm an expert nutritionist and wellness coach. I honestly love what I do, and *whenever* the topics of food, movement, and mindset come up in conversation, I start nerding out with whoever will nerd out with me! It could be when I'm chatting with my Uber driver, when I'm in line at the grocery store, or it's even happened a couple of times in the sauna!

What fascinates me the most with these conversations is that I've noticed that there's a clear difference between genders in how we prefer to do things, whether that's working out or weight loss. The guys seem to favor rigid meal plans and "hustle until you make it" exercise programs that they can follow to the letter, while us ladies tend to prefer a more flexible approach where we tune in and listen to our bodies.

However, the diet and fitness industry *loves* to sell women the guy-centered method. As a result, so many women come to me after trying to follow these very masculine regimes, feeling overwhelmed, demotivated, and like they have failed to stick to the plan perfectly.

Can you relate? If so, I want to make one thing *noticeably clear*: none of this is your fault. The system is not tailored to your fundamental needs as a woman and instead is breeding a ton of self-judgement, shame, and yo-yo dieting.

I love that some health and wellness practitioners are recognizing this and helping women choose forms of nutrition and movement that are aligned with their bodies. The problem I'm seeing increasingly with this is that it's also highly commercialized, especially when it comes to functional medicine.

Most functional medicine practitioners prescribe complicated protocols with a ton of supplements that you must take every single day. To me, this feels a lot like the guy-centered approach I mentioned above, don't you agree?

I studied at one of the top nutrition schools in the UK and have years of experience successfully helping clients feel amazing without piles of pills. Tooting my own horn aside, my point is that I can categorically tell you that most healthy people typically don't need supplements so long as they're eating a balanced diet.

Supplementation is only necessary when our bodies are severely out of balance, which happens in chronic illnesses like cancer, or when we are unable to fully satisfy our bodies' nutritional needs through food, as is the case with eating disorders. Otherwise, food comes first.

For starters, our body utilizes nutrients from food more efficiently than it does from supplements. Then there's the fact that, if we concentrate on supplementation, there is a chance that we will neglect our fundamental eating practices and use supplements to justify unhealthy habits.

On top of this, the supplement industry is unregulated, the quality of supplements varies, and there's just so much out there to choose from. If we're confused over what foods are beneficial for us, imagine how confusing it is to work out what supplements to take!

The functional medicine industry profits from this fact. My client, Gemma, was taking over 60 pills daily under the advice of a functional medicine practitioner. When Gemma told me she was feeling tired and experiencing stomach upsets, I knew what to recommend. Within days of going cold turkey on the supplements, her symptoms disappeared.

Look, I'm not saying that supplementation is *never* useful; for example, in the UK, I'd recommend my clients take a vitamin D supplement during the winter to prevent deficiency because the sun isn't strong enough at that time of year for our bodies to produce enough vitamin D. Meanwhile, taking essential omega-3 fatty acids can be helpful if you don't eat oily fish once or twice per week.

However, don't fall into the trap of feeling like you need to take a whole medicine cabinet just because the holistic health world tells you to. I highly encourage you to give yourself time to consider whether pumping yourself full of pills is part of being in your power and what it might look like instead to trust your body's own wisdom when it comes to providing the nourishment it needs.

To me, we can't be in a place of empowerment if we're not fully rooted in our physical power center; our bodies. Through the process of being told and sold what, when, and how to eat and move, we've lost this vital connection. I totally acknowledge that it's a skill and a practice to be able to go within, listen to what your body is telling you, and choose what to do based on this. But, as you're about to discover, this is possible even if you've spent decades at war with your body.

The Cure

As someone who helps women make peace with food and exercise, and who has been on her own journey to stop calorie counting, over-exercising, and feeling guilty about what she eats, intuitive eating and moving for pleasure, not punishment, are practices near and dear to my heart.

Intuitive eating involves nourishing your body by listening to and acting on your body's signals. No food rules, no calorie counting, no restrictions—just you and your body. Meanwhile, moving for pleasure, not punishment, means tuning into how your body feels and choosing a form of movement based on this that aligns with helping you feel good. It's the way you ate and moved before the diet and fitness industries started telling you what, when, and how to eat and exercise. It's not a matter of learning how to eat intuitively or move for pleasure, but a matter of remembering.

Intuitive eating and moving for pleasure are the most effective ways to empower yourself with your food and exercise choices: you (and only you) get to decide what's best for your body. It's also the fastest route to making peace with food and exercise: having a balanced approach to fueling and moving your body. And get this—it's sustainable and enjoyable!

My clients have experienced a range of benefits, including increased energy, better sleep, and improved athletic performance, sometimes within a matter of weeks of adopting intuitive eating and moving for pleasure.

However, if you're over there reading this and starting to notice a few fears creeping in about trying intuitive eating and moving for pleasure, you're not alone. Something I see a lot of women struggle with, especially all you high achievers out there, is the addiction to pushing yourself to the limit every single time you move. This can make anything else seem pointless, and you ignore your body's request for something gentler.

Take, for example, my friend Becky. At seven months pregnant, Becky was told by her doctor that she needed to stop intense exercise and switch to more restful forms of movement because her baby was in the 15th percentile for size and any smaller would be a health risk. Of course, she dutifully followed the advice, but admitted feeling super uncomfortable "just" doing yoga.

Even when you know some forms of movement are more conducive to caring for your body or your body is sending signals that tell you to take things slower, do you disregard this and want to push on through out of fear that you're not trying hard enough?

With intuitive eating, you may also have the fear that you'll gain weight, or that your symptoms will get worse because you don't have a rigid regime to follow, like calorie counting or supplementation. *"Surely everything will get out of control quickly if I just leave it up to my body?"* I hear you asking.

What you're saying is that you don't trust your body with your food choices. That's because, like most women, you've been taught *not* to trust yourself with anything from an early age, and this has been reinforced repeatedly over time.

I totally understand why it might feel scary to trust your body when you've been battling with it for so long. However, I can't even begin to describe how smart your body really is. It knows what it needs. It's just the diet industry that has convinced you otherwise. The ability to listen to and trust your body is something that can be developed over time and with a few simple tools, some of which I share below.

For now, let's tackle the deeper issue: your fear of losing control. This is yet another illusion created by the diet and fitness industry to keep you stuck in its talons. With intuitive eating and moving for pleasure, you're in fact *gaining* control of your body from diets, calorie counting apps, products, and programs. Where the diet and fitness industries take away your power, intuitive eating and moving for pleasure give it back to you. How freeing is that?

But I get it; it may not feel this way to begin with, and you may feel anxiety, guilt, shame, and judgment around your food and exercise choices. Learning to trust your body and regain healthy control over your food and exercise choices, especially after so long, is a journey, and on any journey, there will always be unknowns.

The key to stepping forward on your journey is to start small and take things one step at a time. This will allow you to expand your comfort zone gradually so, while still a little scary, you don't overactivate your sympathetic nervous system—the part of you that becomes stuck in paralysis or runs away. As with most things, the more you practice, the easier it will get, and the easier it gets, the more you will trust yourself. But to do this, you need to start somewhere.

The Witchual

I've listed my top four ways to explore intuitive eating and moving for pleasure without feeling completely overwhelmed, so that you can reconnect to your body and fully step into your power.

Tune into Your Hunger

It may sound basic, and it is, which is why, for those starting on their intuitive eating journey, rating your hunger on a scale of 1 to 10 and using this to know when to eat as opposed to sticking to a rigid routine, can be powerful. In fact, I've found it so effective for my clients that I featured this technique in my first book, *Reclaim the Rebel*.

Listen to the Signals

Investing the time to understand the language of your body is one of the most priceless gifts you can give to yourself. One method is to rate your level of hunger on a scale of 1 to 10. But occasionally, you might interpret your body's signals incorrectly. For instance, you might mistakenly believe that your body is requesting cookies when it wants something sweet.

Similarly, if you've been under or overnourishing your body for a while, it could be the case that your hunger signals (or lack thereof) aren't always telling you the whole picture, so it's important to get curious about other signals your body is sending, for example; Are your periods missing or irregular? Are you constipated? Is your hair falling out?

Getting curious about the signals your body is sending out is the fastest way to learn your body's unique language. Once you have an idea of what it's trying to tell you, it's important to take the appropriate action, whether that's choosing an apple, eating a cookie, or seeking professional support to re-establish balance in your body. Like any language, it takes practice to master, so show yourself a ton of love and compassion as you learn how to navigate your body's signals.

Ask Yourself Better Questions

To assist you in the process of learning your body's language and acting on what it needs, start asking your body questions. For example, when it comes to moving for pleasure, ask your body how it's feeling today. Does it feel energized and ready to be challenged? Or does it feel a bit sluggish and in need of gentle movement or even complete rest?

It's possible that as you begin to ask these questions, you notice your body feels a little out of balance; maybe your Achilles is extremely tight or your right shoulder has a nagging ache, for instance. Again, get curious about this; your body is attempting to communicate with you. Ask yourself further questions like: "Do I need to spend more time stretching before working out? Is there a need for me to rest and allow my body to heal more in between workouts? What types of movements could I perform to help with this?" Then act upon the answer.

When my client Heather started getting curious about her lower back pain, she stopped neglecting her body after years of ignoring what it was trying to tell her. When she asked the right questions, she effortlessly rediscovered her love of Tai Chi and resolved her back pain within days. She described it as "huge" that she could treat her body with this type of tenderness and care.

Have Some Support

Having support is invaluable on a journey like this because it does take time and inevitably there will be bumps in the road. I highly recommend having a supportive network of friends and family, as well as a coach who knows how to navigate barriers quickly and effectively in your way. This is especially powerful when this person has also walked the path you are taking and can shine a light into the unknown. I'll be talking more about support networks in Steps 7 (Brace for the Witch Slap) and 8 (End of the Battle of the Hexes).

The Wisdom

For now, I invite you to turn inward and re-establish your connection with your incredibly wise inner GPS regarding your food and workout choices. This is not a one-and-done thing; it's a practice that requires patience, self-compassion, and a suite of tools, some of which I've shared in this section. Discover more of these tools so that you can learn to trust your body even if you've spent decades at war with it by heading to www.reclaimthewitch.com.

STEP 4: GET *PsCyclic*

The Curse

As you discovered in the last section, learning to listen to and act on what your body is telling you is an essential part of unlocking your power. After all, your body is your power center. But it's not a linear, single-mode power center. Instead, women are naturally cyclic; physically, physiologically, emotionally, and energetically.

The best example of this is our menstrual cycle; between the ages of around 12 and 52[6] our hormones ebb and flow over approximately 28 days, and consequently so too do our emotions, energy levels, appetite, strength, and stamina – to name but a few.[7]

However, we're taught from an incredibly early age by the patriarchy to suppress this natural cycle. For example, feminine hygiene commercials make us feel like we need to hide our periods and hustle through them in tight white jeans. Have you noticed they also try to sanitize the whole experience by using blue water to represent our blood? No wonder many women nowadays view their period as a major annoyance, slightly gross, and something that should be talked about in hushed and apologetic tones. Maybe you can relate?

However, have you fully considered how powerful your period (or the potential to have one in your lifetime) really is? I'm not talking about the "boss babe" and "superwomen" stereotypes that are shoved in our faces by advertisers. I'm talking about the fact that having a period means you can create life. That, sister, is power! And the patriarchy wants to control it by controlling you and your body. It does this by creating a disempowering system for how we treat our bodies, and the lack of education we receive about our bodies.

A few lessons on the physiological aspects of the reproductive cycle were taught to most of us in school, but we were never really sat down and told how this practically applied to our lives (aside from the fact that we could use pads or tampons when we bled and that we could use contraceptives to prevent getting pregnant).

Personally, I had never even considered whether the things that had been suggested to me—including the artificially scented sanitary products and IUD—were healthy for my body. This resulted in several issues, including an agonizing experience at the doctor, where my womb rejected the IUD, and I passed out from the pain.

Ladies, I know I'm not the only one here who was just "going along with things." Let's get super honest here: How many of you merely took the pill because your doctor prescribed it or used tampons because your friends did?

There's no shame or judgement if you have used or continue to use these. I was on hormonal birth control for over a decade because I thought it meant I could keep hustling through life without worrying about irregular periods or acne breakouts, when in fact it was simply a band-aid for me not properly looking after myself.

After I recovered from my 10-year battle with anorexia and developed osteoporosis by the age of 23, nurturing my body became one of my highest values. After a lot of research and reading, I realized that taking hormonal contraceptives was not conducive to honoring this value or being fully in my power. It was a very personal decision to come off hormonal birth control, and I am by no means saying that you should too.

However, what I *am* saying is that most of us lacked educators or parents who were knowledgeable or confident enough to discuss the power of women's bodies and how we could honor this power in a way that felt good for us.

Again, it makes total sense that we find it awkward to talk about our menstrual cycle, view it as a big inconvenience, and succumb to the misleading marketing of feminine hygiene products that encourage us to hide our periods.

Instead of honoring our cycle, many of us push on through despite being curled over with excruciating cramps and undeniable food cravings, while trying as hard as we can to hide our emotions to look normal (whatever the hell that is)! But, in doing this, we ignore our feminine essence and what we're meant to feel, express, and learn from.

Our mental and physical health is suffering as a result; fertility and reproductive issues are at an all-time high, and women come to me burned out and exhausted from overworking and stuffing their emotions down out of fear of being seen by others as too much, unstable, or crazy.

Take, for example, my client Gabby, a mom of three young kids, business owner, and all-round amazing woman. She told me when we first began working together that she had broken down in tears during a business meeting the week before and still felt extremely embarrassed about it. We determined that she had been hustling along at work and home, spinning all the plates, for months. Even though she made every effort to conceal her exhaustion, she had to cry to diffuse some of the pressure she'd been putting on herself.

The mental and physical toll of trying to suppress your emotions and ignore your body's cyclic nature is significant. For example, it can reinforce low self-worth, perfectionism, and people-pleasing, as well as disrupt your sleep and drain you of energy. Ultimately, it sabotages your relationship with yourself and your body because you can never reach the unrealistic standards you've set for yourself and, as a result, always feel you're lacking in something. You might turn to social media, food and alcohol, shopping, and personal development programs to find the answer to what you're missing.

And when you don't? You move on to the next thing. If this sounds familiar, I know how you feel. Honestly, I did the same until I realized I was already 'whole' and what I *really* craved was the connection I'd lost with my body and the cyclic feminine power held within her via years of societal conditioning, BS (beliefs and stories), and self-abusive behaviors I thought were helping me "succeed" in my health, career, and relationships.

Over the last couple of years, I've met so many high-achieving women just like you and me who, deep-down, long to reconnect with our cycles and the magic held within our incredible female bodies.

The Cure

Before the patriarchy, women would gather in ceremonial circles under the new moon to celebrate their bleed. It was considered a sacred time when women had heightened intuition and could more easily communicate with the divine. The whole community fully embraced women's PsCyclic nature and the close relationship between the moon and the feminine.

It's no coincidence that our menstrual cycle and the moon cycle are both roughly 28 days in length. Just like the moon, every month we go through our own phases of waxing, fullness, waning, and renewing. How amazing and magical is that? This also applies to women who, for whatever reason, do not bleed.

In the table below, I've outlined how the four phases of the menstrual cycle map against the four phases of the moon.

Moon Phase	What's happening with the moon	Menstrual Phase (approximate days in your cycle)	What's happening within your body
New	The moon isn't visible in the sky.	Menstruation/ Period (approximately days 1-7)	Your estrogen and progesterone levels are at their lowest. If you're not pregnant, you shed the lining of your womb, ready to start a new cycle. You may feel like "hiding" from the world at this point in your cycle.
Waxing	Over the next 14 days, the moon grows larger in the sky.	Pre-ovulation/ Follicular (approximately days 7-13)	After your period, your estrogen and FSH (Follicle-Stimulating Hormone) levels start to rise, and your energy levels begin to increase.
Full	The moon appears as a complete circle in the sky.	Ovulation (approximately days 14-20)	Your estrogen level is at its highest, and LH (Luteinizing Hormone) spikes, causing an egg to be released from your ovaries. You'll likely feel at your brightest at this point in your cycle.
Waning	Over the next 14 days, the moon starts to disappear again.	Pre-menstruation/ Luteal (approximately days 21-28)	Progesterone levels rise in preparation for a potential pregnancy. However, if that egg released during ovulation hasn't been fertilized, your estrogen and progesterone levels begin to dip, and as a result, so do your energy levels (and potentially your tolerance for BS!).

If you've gone through menopause, are on hormonal birth control, or for any other reason do not experience a menstrual cycle, use this table to consider other ways your body cycles with the moon. For example, maybe you notice that your energy levels increase as the moon waxes, peak at the full moon, and then decrease as the moon wanes.

Historically, most women bled on the new moon, but modern living means that most of us do not. If that's the case for you, please know that this doesn't make you any less powerful or magical, so don't use this as another excuse to hate your body. Regardless of where the moon is in her cycle, use the table above to consider how each phase of your cycle symbolizes each phase of the moon.

The days listed in this table are also approximations because each woman's cycle is slightly different. What's normal for me is likely different from what's normal for you. That's why it's so important to become familiar with *your* cycle and what normal specifically looks like for *you*.

Since coming off hormonal contraception and becoming familiar with and observing my cycle, I've gained an intimate understanding of how my body uniquely ebbs and flows over the course of a month, and in turn, I can predict when I'll feel more sociable, when I'll need more rest, and when I'll crave more chocolate. This has elevated me to a whole new level of inner confidence and kindness toward my body.

It's also made me a better nutritionist and wellness coach. First, I can schedule my work to fit around my strengths at various times of the month. And second, it's encouraged me to give personalized nutrition and movement recommendations to support my clients' menstrual cycle and address any hormonal imbalances that lead to painful periods, breakouts, and bloating so that they can reclaim confidence in their incredible female bodies.

To be completely honest, when I first opened Nutrition by Lizzy, I preferred working with male clients. Getting them results was so easy due to their more predictable physiology. Give a man something like intermittent fasting, low fat, low carb, or HIIT, and they'll most likely see results quickly.

However, female bodies are fundamentally different from male bodies. For example, intermittent fasting can cause menstrual periods to suspend until normal eating patterns are restored.[8]

Women in their reproductive years should avoid intermittent fasting, especially if they have issues with fertility or are trying to conceive. Most trainers and nutrition gurus don't account for these unique factors or the natural physical changes that women's bodies go through over the course of a month as well as a lifetime.

They also don't account for your feminine need for flexibility in building and maintaining habits. We always hear how consistency is key to forming healthy habits, don't we? I even talked about this in *Reclaim the Rebel*. But honestly, that's just half the story. Consistency *does* have a role, but we also need to recognize that, due to our cyclic nature, there may be times when we are inconsistent, and that's okay. The trick is to align your actions in the present with whatever is in your body's best interests.

For instance, suppose you were training for a 10K run but missed the gym one week because you were on your period. Because you are aware that you require more rest during this time and are confident that you will resume training as soon as your body is prepared, this lack of consistency is not a problem. This level of intimate body awareness is empowering, instills a quiet confidence in your own abilities, and ultimately represents a step closer to embracing your inner witch.

The Witchual

Everybody is different, so please do not approach your cycle the same way as me (or anyone else). I only work with clients on a one-to-one basis because I want to understand you, your body, your lifestyle, and your current struggles. This means I can give you fully personalized nutrition and workout recommendations so that you work with your body, not against it, and reach your goals without feeling defeated or deprived. If this sounds good to you, visit www.reclaimthewitch.com to find out more.

In the meantime, grab a journal (it can be as fancy or as plain as you like) or turn to the journal section at the back of this book, and start becoming familiar with your cycle by tracking how you feel on a day-to-day basis. Write down anything from one word to a whole page to describe your mood (tired, reactive, relaxed, happy, anxious), how your body feels (achy, tender, energized, sluggish), and your eating habits (hungry, full, craving chocolate). If you menstruate, keep track of where you are in your cycle.

I like to track how my cycle aligns with the moon cycle, so when I journal, I also note what sign and phase the moon is in. This isn't essential, but if you do decide to go all in with this, you'll get *so* much intel on yourself and your body. And, as we know, knowledge is power. To find out what phase and sign the moon is in, I use AstroSeek.com. I like their moon calendar because the information is clearly displayed, and you can adjust it to your precise geographic location.

For ease, I write my cycle journal underneath my dream journal every morning. Here's an example:

> January 24th, 2023: Woke up super hungry, body aches a little, boobs feel a bit tender. Pre-menstruation, day 23. Waxing moon in Pisces.
>
> January 25th, 2023: Feeling a bit all over the place and angry with the world. Distinct 'fuck it' vibes! Pre-menstruation, day 24. Waxing moon in Aries.

After several months of doing this for yourself, you'll likely start to notice patterns. For example, in how your body physically feels, when you have cravings, and how much energy you have at different points in your cycle. Once you start noticing these patterns, you can start to create personal practices and rituals to support yourself as you ebb and flow through your cycle.

Again, these will be unique to you, and if you're looking for guidance to optimize your workouts and nutrition, please seek personalized advice from an expert who is familiar with women's unique physiology. Don't just go on Instagram or YouTube and hope for the best. Not everyone is the same, and you need a professional who can look at the whole picture for you.

While this is not to be taken as advice specifically for you or as a substitute for professional support, I want to help get you started. That's why below I've included a couple of my favorite ways to honor what most women find the most challenging parts of their cycle: the waning and renewing phases (i.e., pre-menstruation and menstruation, if you have a menstrual cycle).

Eat the Good Stuff

During my "I-need-chocolate-NOW" pre-menstruation phase, I listen to my craving. Acting on cravings doesn't have to mean making unhealthy choices, as I want to show you with the following delicious and hassle-free cacao hot chocolate recipe.

Cacao Hot Chocolate

Ingredients:

▽ 1 cup of a milk of your choice (I use 2% dairy milk)
▽ 1 tablespoon of raw cacao powder
▽ 1 tablespoon of local honey (you can also use maple syrup)
▽ 1/4 teaspoon vanilla extract
▽ Optional: 1/2 teaspoon ground cinnamon

Instructions:

1. Combine all the ingredients into a saucepan over high heat, using a whisk to break up any clumps.

2. Keep stirring until smooth and piping hot, then pour into a mug and serve warm.

3. Top with extras such as shaved chocolate, if desired.

Rest and Regenerate

I give myself time to slow down, nest, and rest during my period. This may seem indulgent and uncomfortable, especially for women who are doers and set the bar for themselves unrealistically high. Trust me; I've been there. If you've read *Reclaim the Rebel*, you'll know this only led to exhaustion and burnout.

Resting physically and mentally is so important during this part of your cycle. You aren't meant to be constantly productive, and in trying to push on through, you're harming your body and setting yourself up to burn out physically and emotionally. Stop "do-doing" on yourself. Let yourself have breaks in your workday, go to bed earlier, and say "no" to work projects and social engagements if they don't feel aligned with you taking care of yourself.

The latter has been particularly challenging for me; as a recovered people-pleaser, I always felt guilty for expressing my needs, especially when I knew someone wanted something different from me. But again, this is all part of shedding that self-suppression I mentioned earlier and stepping into our feminine power. I'm not going to lie and say it's always easy, but it *is* necessary. The more we practice, the easier it gets. The easier it gets, the more we disown the fears about being the bitch/selfish/crazy lady and give these stories back to their original owners (more on this in the next step).

The Wisdom

Most women have been led to believe that we need to do things just like men, including how, what, and when we workout and eat. However, we are different from them— physically, physiologically, emotionally, and energetically. Women are naturally cyclic. This means all those conventional plans and regimes aren't going to work for you in the same way they would for a man.

Instead, you need to foster a way of nurturing yourself that works with your unique female body. I've provided suggestions above so that you can start doing this for yourself, but I also appreciate that you're busy and may not have the time to research and create practices that best suit you. That's why I offer a set of personalized nutrition and movement recommendations for my clients so that you can confidently step into the body you love with ease. Visit www.reclaimthewitch.com to claim yours.

STEP 5: *Spell* IT OUT

The Curse

My favorite quote of all time belongs to Florence Scovel Shinn: "*Your word is your wand.*" It always reminds me how the words we speak, think, and write are powerful spells that create our reality.

In addition to being extremely potent, it's also rather poetic that what is thought of as the most typical trait of being a witch—aside from the pointy nose, cackle, and warts (sigh…thanks Hollywood)—comes so naturally to us all: using our words to "spell" something into existence.

We can use them as a tool to manifest the outcomes we want for ourselves. We can also (often unknowingly) become spellbound, where we use words to curse ourselves and create a negative feedback loop of undesirable outcomes.

In my private practice, I often hear women talk about their bodies in a way they would *never* talk about someone else's. I've heard everything from general "I'm so ugly/fat/disgusting" remarks to specific criticism of individual body parts; my client Hannah used to say, "My boobs are so saggy; they look like my grandmother's." Can you relate? Have you ever talked to your body in a negative way?

If you've read *Reclaim the Rebel*, you'll know I refer to this as our "inner mean girl." She creates a distorted body image when we look in the mirror, have our photos taken, and get dressed every morning. She also creates a distorted self-image through the unhelpful beliefs passed on to us by other people, marketing, and unattainable societal standards created by the patriarchy. The longer our inner mean girl is in charge, the harder it becomes to break the spells that keep us stuck.

For this reason, I'm very mindful of the words I use when it comes to my body, but also my overall health and wellness, as well as my relationships, career, and finances. For example, I've put "try," "struggle," and "should" in my personal word jail because they feel so disempowering.

I've also become wary of the idea of "becoming your best," which is used a lot in the personal development industry. It's such an appealing concept, isn't it? But in the process of chasing this, you're subconsciously saying you don't feel "good enough" as you are, that you're lacking in something, or that you're "broken."

As a result, you ignore your own wisdom because you no longer trust that you know yourself better than anyone else does. You look outside yourself for the answers and waste time and money on personal development courses and "feel better" programs, and when nothing works, you seek the next thing. It can feel like an addition.

The workings of our inner mean girl and her words are often subtle but potent in keeping us trapped. Luckily, alongside our inner mean girl, we also have an inner witch who can transmute the spells that prevent us from fully stepping into our power. The first step in this is becoming aware of our inner mean girl voice and where in our lives we are currently spellbound.

Head to the journal section at the back of this book and take a moment to jot down a list of things you notice yourself routinely thinking and saying—your spells. Then, consider:

▽ What are the outcomes of these spells?
▽ Do you know where these came from?
▽ Are they true? Or are they just subjective interpretations?
▽ Are they yours, or have they just been passed on to you by someone else?

When you do this, you'll probably start to notice where you're being kept spellbound and how this is preventing you from fully stepping into your power.

Let's revisit the story I introduced at the beginning of this book as an example. The reactions of that little girl on the playground and my grandparents created the subconscious spell that "being myself is not okay." Although this is obviously untrue, it kept me from feeling secure in who I was and from being able to help other women step into their most powerful, authentic selves and truly love their bodies.

If you're like most people, it's likely a lot of your spells originated in childhood before the age of eight, which is when you start to develop critical thinking skills, become aware of different perspectives, and form your own point of view.[9]

Up until that point, your brain's architecture is still developing, so any spells will easily become etched in your subconscious.[10]

This means it can be difficult to even recognize that they're there. However, don't stress about what you can't see. Start with the spells you *are* aware of and go from there. The more you practice awareness, the more you will reveal old spells you never realized you were holding onto, and the more you will be able to free yourself from their grip.

The Cure

You can probably imagine how letting go of these old spells can completely change your life. Not only does it release you from other people's curses and provide you with more freedom and peace, but it also gives you space to create new, more empowering spells.

So, let me ask you this: What new spells could you create that are more aligned with how you want to feel and the life you want to create for yourself?

Imagine the type of person who is fully in her power, and ask yourself what spells she uses. Then, go to the journal pages in the back of this book and re-write a more empowering version for each of the spells that you identified as having you spellbound.

These new spells need to feel realistic and believable so that your subconscious doesn't immediately reject them. So, for example, if your current spell is "My postpartum stretch marks are so ugly," you might want to consider changing it to "My stretch marks are a sign of how incredible my body is to have carried and nourished a little human inside it for 9 months'." You don't have to say, "My body is perfect, and I love my stretch marks," if it doesn't feel good to you. If it does, great. But you don't need to go from 0 to 60 immediately; if you can choose a spell that makes you feel just a tiny bit better than the old one does, that's enough.

Now that you're aware of where you've been spellbound and have new empowering spells to replace the old and disempowering ones, the key is to practice replacing the old with the new every time they come up. At first, it may take a little more effort, and you'll need to give yourself some self-compassion as you learn to do this, but as with any practice, it gets easier and more efficient over time. You'll start to notice that you're gradually releasing yourself from other people's curses and naturally choosing increased spells that align with how you want to feel and who you want to be as a woman fully in her power.

STEP 5: SPELL IT OUT

The Witchual

As I've mentioned in previous steps, it's important that you work with both your conscious and subconscious when reclaiming your inner witch. Think of the subconscious as the lock and the conscious as the key to your power. You can only unlock your power when your conscious actions align with the subconscious part of your brain. Below, I've listed some ways in which you can do this to effectively transmute your spells.

I highly encourage you to focus on one spell at a time and to make sure you have a clear intention before you begin; What is the spell you're letting go of? What is your new spell? And how do you want to feel about this new spell?

Sticky Notes

Once you have this clear, one of my favorite ways to transmute a spell is to write your old spell on a sticky note, rip it up, and throw it away. Then, write your new spell on another set of sticky notes, and put them somewhere (such as above your desk or on your mirror) where you will see them often and therefore read them automatically. Replace your post-it notes when you notice a spell has been effectively transmuted.

Crystals and Jewelry

Enchanting an object, such as jewelry or crystals, with your new spell is an alternative, more symbolic way to work with spells. Before doing this, make sure you cleanse any negative energy from the object. For example, you could put it out on the night of a full moon. When you're ready, hold the object in your hand, close your eyes, and put your brain and body into a relaxed state by breathing deeply.

As I mentioned in Step 2: S-witch On Your Powers, I like to use a technique called box breathing to slow my brainwaves down and activate my parasympathetic nervous system—the one that tells your body to rest and digest. Try box breathing: breathe in for a count of four, hold for a count of four, breathe out for a count of four, and pause for a count of four. Repeat for two minutes to get your body and brain into a relaxed state and access your subconscious.

Now that you've got access to your subconscious, declare your new spell and take a moment to focus on how it makes you feel. Then, imagine pushing the spell from your mind down through your neck, shoulders, and arms, into your fingers, and out into the object. When you're finished, open your eyes.

Once you enchant an object, you can carry it around with you or place it on your altar (see Step 9: Be a Wand-erer).

Candles

Candles represent the element of fire, which symbolizes transformation, so candle magic is perfect for when you want to transmute your spells. You could use a candle to burn your old spells instead of ripping them up; of course, practice fire safety while you do this.

Alternatively, enchant a candle in the same way you would a piece of jewelry or crystal. Just make sure you use an unused (and unlit) candle whenever you infuse it with a new spell. The spell will be activated each time you burn the candle.

You can also go one step further and choose a candle in a color that represents the type of spell you're focusing on; for example, a green candle can be used for money spells, a pink candle for relationship spells, and a white candle for inner peace and harmony spells. Head to www.reclaimthewitch.com for a printable worksheet of different candle color meanings.

Water

If fire and rocks aren't your thing, another powerful element to work with is water (especially if your new spell carries a lot of emotional charge). Pour a glass of water and go through the same process of closing your eyes and sending your spell from your mind into the water. The spell will then be activated as you drink the water.

Moon Water

Every month I make moon water. On the night of a full moon, I fill a glass mason jar with filtered tap water, put its lid on, go through the above process of infusing my new spell into the water, and place the jar on my outdoor altar to be bathed in moonlight. In the morning, I store the jar in the fridge to be used for spell work.

Other witches do it slightly differently and put a post-it note with the spell they want to infuse into the water under the jar as the water is being charged overnight. As with all the tools I share in this book, the most important thing is to experiment, have fun, and do what feels best for you.

The Wisdom

The words we think, speak, and write are powerful spells; if used carelessly, they can keep us spellbound. In this step, I walk your inner witch through the process of recognizing the spells that limit you and transmuting them into spells that align with how you want to feel and who you want to be as a woman fully in her power. As you play with the tools I've shared, take photos and tag me on Instagram @nutritionbylizzy; I'll send you a spell-cial gift so that you can have even more fun transmuting your spells!

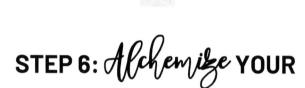

STEP 6: *Alchemize* YOUR

INTERPRETATION

The Curse

All this talk of spells, enchantments, moon water, and manifestations may leave you wondering, "Is this real, or is it all in my head?"

If so, you're not alone. I've asked myself this question *many* times on my journey to reclaiming my inner witch. But then I follow this with another question: "Does it matter?" My answer is always a resounding "No!"

That's because choosing to believe in my magic, your magic, and everyone else's magic makes me feel so much joy and feeds my curiosity, which in turn leaves me open to the wonder of life and all that is possible.

I've also experienced so much, both in my dreams and in my waking life, that believing in the immense power housed within each one of us is a complete no-brainer for me.

During an energy clearing session (of which I've done many), I suddenly had a vision of an ice cream scoop scraping out gunk from inside my intestines and stomach. When I told the practitioner about this, she encouraged me to stay focused and remain curious about what was happening.

Soon after the appointment ended, I started feeling *intense* soreness in my abdomen. I could barely sit upright. I hadn't done an ab workout, eaten anything odd that day, or had any digestive issues. The only thing different was the ice cream scoop I'd encountered in this energy clearing session.

The pain in my abdomen went away as quickly as it came, and I still don't know for certain what caused it. However, my intuitive interpretation that I was removing a ton of energetic gunk from my body during that session was enough and, to this day, continues to be, the only thing I need to choose to believe in magic.

What will it take for *you* to choose to believe in magic?

The Cure

Having doubts about the validity and reality of your experiences is completely normal.

With two science degrees, I've been trained to use quantitative data to evaluate and make objective sense of the world. However, in the cases of intuition, magic, and manifestation, this type of data is often unavailable, and instead we must rely on our subjective interpretation.

This can feel super uncomfortable, especially if, like me, you're a fan of logic, reasoning, statistics, and always having a definitive answer. I see you, my friend; stay with me here. I'm not asking you to completely throw logic and reasoning out the window; they have a key role in discerning real from fake in both scientific and magical matters. All I ask is for you to fully consider your interpretations.

For example:

▽ What if there are some things that cannot be explained by numbers?
▽ What if science doesn't have all the answers?
▽ What if there is no correct answer?
▽ What if part of life is unexplainable?
▽ What if magic lived all around us, and within us?

Finding magic in the everyday depends entirely on your interpretations and which of these you choose to believe; from the "big" experience that completely stops you in your tracks to smaller ones that turn the corners of your mouth into a little smile.

The truth is, there are many potential interpretations for every experience we have in life, from how we interpret what someone says to us to how we interpret our reflection in the mirror. To demonstrate my point, I want you to take a moment and write down five different interpretations that you can think of as to why I chose to eat oatmeal as opposed to yogurt for breakfast this morning.

Here are my five interpretations:

1. It was cold outside today, and I wanted something warm to eat
2. Oatmeal is healthier than yogurt
3. Oatmeal is more filling than yogurt
4. I didn't have any yogurt in my fridge, so I had to choose oatmeal
5. I went running this morning, so needed the carbohydrates to fuel my workout

Now, I rattled those different interpretations out in less than 30 seconds, and each could be correct. But how would you know which one is which? And could all five be true? You could look at scientific studies on the health benefits of yogurt versus oatmeal, or you could look at what the temperature was this morning in Los Angeles. But you cannot know just by using quantitative data and traditional science.

The same goes for anything magical. Let's take the example of my experience with the ice cream scoop. Can you think of five interpretations of what happened?

Here are mine:

1. The session cleared energetic blocks in my body, and I experienced them through the imagery of an ice cream scoop

2. Lying down for that long is boring, so my brain started making up images to keep me distracted

3. I was hungry, and so I started to think of ice cream

4. When I was picturing the ice cream scoop digging around my belly, my abs started to contract, and that's what gave me the soreness after the session

5. I'm a little bonkers and have an active imagination

Maybe one or all of these interpretations are true. But again, how would we know? It's not a matter of necessarily finding the correct answer but of choosing an interpretation and trusting the accuracy of that choice.

Trusting our interpretation is something a lot of us struggle with, especially when it comes to magic. That's because the patriarchy wants us to doubt ourselves so that it can continue to control and suppress our power. One way they try to do this is by waving their own spells about being crazy for believing in magic and smart for believing in science.

But are science and magic mutually exclusive? I'd argue they don't have to be. Consider, for example, how advances in technology have meant we can now fly across the Atlantic and even turn lead into gold.[11]

What would your great-great grandparents say to *that*? Scientific tools and knowledge have enabled us to accomplish many things that were once thought impossible. That's magic right there.

The Witchual

If scientists can alchemize your interpretation of what's possible, so can you. The key is learning to trust your interpretations. My favorite way to build more confidence in my interpretations when it comes to magical matters is through divination tools such as pendulums, tarot cards, and oracle cards.

Using a Pendulum (AKA Dowsing)

A pendulum is a divination tool that is frequently (but not always) made of a crystal and can help you decide on issues relating to everything from your finances to your health. They come in a variety of materials and designs and are available in most esoteric stores as well as online.

Before using your pendulum for the first time, cleanse its energy either by leaving it out overnight under a full moon or via a technique known as smudging, where you burn a type of sacred herb or resin and waft the smoke around you, your objects, and your environment to clear the energies (see Step 9: Be a Wand-erer for more details).

The next step is to calibrate your pendulum by holding it in one hand and asking it to show you what "yes" is. Then ask it to show you what "no" is. You'll notice the pendulum moving in a certain way for the "yes" and in another way for the "no." Remember what these different movements are and what answer they correspond to.

Alternatively, you can calibrate your pendulum by asking it some yes-or-no questions that you already know the answer to, for example, "Is my name Lizzy Cangro?" or "Do I like chocolate?" or "Is my favorite color blue?" Then take note of the different movements that the "yes" and "no" answers produce.

Once you've done this, you're ready to ask your pendulum some yes-or-no questions that you want to find the answer to, such as, "Is this new business idea something to pursue?" or "Is this new relationship a good fit for me?"

Tarot and Oracle Cards

My preferred divination methods are tarot and oracle cards. Tarot cards have more traditional meanings and a specific deck size. On the other hand, there are many different themes and sizes for the decks of oracle cards. I enjoy using both and purchasing decks that I feel intuitively drawn to.

Before the first use, I'll clear the energy of my cards just as I described above with the pendulum. This is crucial because, before they reach you or me, tools like these have likely been handled by numerous people. We want to get rid of any lingering negative energy that they may have picked up in this process.

When I'm ready to use my cards, I shuffle the deck and, in my head, ask the cards a question I want clarity on. I'll shuffle until one (or more) cards jump out at me. Not everyone pulls their cards like this, but I've come to realize that's how my cards communicate with me.

Other witches might shuffle a certain number of times before drawing a card. Some may draw multiple cards; three (one for your past, one for your present, and one for your future) seems to be a common spread, but I've seen some witches use a lot more. It's entirely up to you.

It's also entirely up to you how frequently you use your cards. Rituals don't need to be rigid. In fact, the word "rigid" is just so, well, rigid. (Remember in the last section I was saying our words matter?) To me, it feels restrictive to have to draw a card on a set schedule, whether that's daily, weekly, or monthly. Instead, I pull a card (or four) whenever I feel like it.

Once you have pulled your card(s), get curious about the images and words you see on the card(s). Just as with dream interpretation, I highly recommend refraining from heading straight to an online dictionary or guidebook. Instead, consider your associations with the images and words on the cards and how they relate to what you asked the cards to show you.

It may come instantly, or it may be something you need to let sit for a while, but you'll know you have an accurate interpretation when you have the all-knowing feeling I talked about earlier and your head isn't getting in the way.

Once you have finished asking your pendulum questions and interpreting your cards, the final step is to make sure you act on the answers you receive. For example, maybe the oracle card you pulled today suggests that you slow down and rest. As a result, you could block some time in your evening to take a nice, long bath and go to bed early. Or maybe you decide to take a vacation. Trust that the guidance you receive and the actions you take are meant for you. The more you do this, the more you will trust in your interpretations…and your magic.

The Wisdom

At some point on your journey to reclaiming your inner witch, you may start questioning whether you really *are* magic. What you're really saying here is that you don't trust your interpretation of the experiences you're having as you unlock your power. This trust is something that is developed over time and with practice.

Some of my favorite tools to help you trust your interpretations include pendulums, tarot cards, and oracle cards. In fact, I've even created a set of oracle cards to accompany *Reclaim the Witch*. Head to www.reclaimthewitch.com and get your hands on these limited-edition cards.

STEP 7: BRACE FOR THE *witch* SLAP

The Curse

In the process of alchemizing your interpretations and reclaiming your magic, your relationships will likely change, both personal and professional, which, if you're anything like me, can feel scary. This is very natural and understandable considering how witches (i.e., women in their power) have been persecuted for centuries.

It's well-known across history and cultures that any woman who refuses to be controlled or suppressed and instead boldly embraces her power, becomes a prime target for the patriarchy and its desperate attempts to slap her back into line.

They might use overt tactics such as publicly attacking a woman's character, body, or both. Take, for example, Adele, who, despite having a *very* successful music career, has been repeatedly criticized about her body.[12] Then there's Taylor Swift, who was criticized for "fat shaming" in one of her music videos when in fact she was just expressing her personal experience of struggling with body image issues.[13]

I'm shocked and deeply saddened whenever I read the social media comments that accompany these types of stories. That's because they highlight a more covetous and arguably dangerous tactic the patriarchy tries to use to control us, turning women against other women. During the witch trials across North America and Europe in the 15th, 16th, and 17th centuries, women were forced to betray one another in fear for their lives.[14]

Nowadays, this has evolved into social media bitch fests and overdramatized stories in gossip magazines about celebrity women arguing over money and men. But it doesn't just affect the rich and famous. In fact, a lot of my clients struggle with comparing themselves and feeling like they need to compete with other women in their daily lives. Can you relate?

If so, it's likely you've inherited this from your mother or grandmother. Most women have accumulated a huge amount of distrust toward one another and fear of stepping into their power over multiple generations. Not only is this recorded in historical documents, but it is also within our DNA.

The famous cherry blossom study in 2013 showed that trauma can be passed down through multiple generations via epigenetics. Neuroscientists at Emory University taught mice to fear the smell of cherry blossoms by associating the scent with mild electric shocks. When they bred these mice, the researchers found the offspring became fearful when they were exposed to the smell, despite never receiving the electric shocks their parents experienced. They were even born with more neurons in their noses and space in their brains devoted to cherry-blossom-smelling. Similar results were then found in their offspring.[15]

We are the product of multiple generations of trauma, just like the mice in the cherry blossom experiment. Only our trauma isn't caused by electric shocks; it's the persecution of powerful women.

The idea of wallowing in victimhood feels yucky to me, so let's not go there. However, it's helpful to understand what's happened to women in the past so that we can treat ourselves and each other with more compassion and realize that the fears we experience today run deep and are widespread. You are not alone, sister. Read that again: you are not alone.

The most common fear as you reclaim your power and fully own your status as a witch is that you will be judged by others. For example, they'll think you're crazy, they'll reject you, or they'll not take you seriously.

When I was 16 years old, my boyfriend made fun of me for showing an interest in astrology; he said it wasn't scientific. As we now know from Step 6: Alchemize Your Interpretation, science and magic aren't separate. However, at the time, I was afraid that he wouldn't love me or that I wouldn't make it as a successful scientist if I pursued my esoteric interests.

Have you ever been, or are you worried about being, judged like this? If so, it can keep you stuck in multiple ways. In my case, it meant I didn't follow my interests, I stayed in my spiritual closet, I didn't seek guidance in unlocking my magic, and I remained trapped by the fear of judgment until my thirties. How is the fear of being judged affecting *you*?

Maybe you've already shed a lot of fear about being judged. If so, great. As you've progressed beyond this and moved further along on your journey of stepping into your power, you may have also noticed several *more* fears come up. For example, as you free yourself from being spellbound (as per Step 5: Spell it Out), you'll likely notice your beliefs and perspective change. With this, you may start to worry about becoming disconnected from those you are close to who remain spellbound, such as your family, friends, and partner. Maybe you fear becoming "too much" or overbearing now that you are expressing yourself more freely. Maybe you're fearful that you'll lose clients.

Whatever fears are coming up for you, it's perfectly natural; fear is a subconscious survival mechanism and becomes super important in certain situations. It's especially helpful when you're nose-to-nose with a lion and need to run away! So, it's not a matter of getting rid of fear completely but of knowing how to move through it when it's limiting you or keeping you trapped in disempowering situations, behaviors, and thoughts.

The Cure

The greatest gift we can give ourselves and the people with whom we are in a relationship (whether that's a friendship, a romantic relationship, a business relationship, etc.) is to show up authentically. This creates deep connections with others and crushes the fear of judgment right in its tracks.

Being authentic requires the courage to be vulnerable, and this courage comes with practice. It's no longer the Middle Ages, and, in the Western world, most women are fortunate that their lives are not at risk if we choose to fully step into our power. Therefore, I strongly encourage you to take some deep breaths (remember how, in Step 2: Switch On Your Powers, I said this was helpful in regulating our nervous system?) and start having more open and vulnerable conversations with those with whom you feel most comfortable doing so. For example, your partner, friends, or family. The more you do this, the easier it will become to authentically share yourself (including your inner witch).

When you're ready to do this publicly, make a post or go "live" on Instagram about your journey so far, including reading this book. While you're at it, tag me @nutritionbylizzy for extra support and high fives.

To my surprise, the world didn't end when I had the courage to share my esoteric side. In fact, while my relationships *did* change, they became deeper and more interesting. As I revealed more of my inner witch, it seemed to give others permission to do the same and share their unique experiences. I was pleasantly surprised that my mum was open to talking about astrology. When I shared my natal astrological chart reading with her, she told me she had encountered a psychic many years before who had predicted similar things to what was in my chart. Pretty cool, right?

Now, I'm not saying that everyone who you talk to will suddenly reveal their spiritual beliefs and experiences, and that's ok. The goal is more about creating space to be authentic and connect with other women (and men; more on this in the next section).

It also allows you to sort through your current relationships, turning your back on those that are not aligned with your being in your power and nurturing those that do feel aligned. By noticing who you genuinely feel uplifted being around versus who feels like an emotional vampire, you'll find it's easier to say "yes" to the people and experiences that are meant for you and "no" to those that suck the life force from you.

Setting boundaries around what I will and won't accept, especially without feeling guilty or judging myself or others, has taken me *years* of practice. It means that some friendships have waned, or I've had to let go of them completely. I've realized that this is not a commentary on me or the other person. It's simply a process of alignment, which is healthy and helpful for everyone involved.

Any time you want to grow, it's crucial to create a community of people you feel aligned with and supported by—what I call your "cheer squad" in *Reclaim the Rebel*. That's because your cheer squad will be there for you in both happy and challenging times to encourage and inspire you to keep going.

I've been lucky enough to have an incredible cheer squad of women and men, who have (quite literally) laughed and cried with me along my journey. However, as someone who grew up with a huge distrust of other women, it's been especially transformative to find a group of women with whom I feel understood, seen, and safe. In my squad, there's room for everyone—no comparison, competition, or drama.

It's so uplifting, especially during the more challenging times, to allow yourself to be held by people like this whom you trust and respect. I'm in massive gratitude to Patty Dominguez and the eight other female entrepreneurs who supported me when I realized that I needed to write this book. I was terrified because I knew I'd be revealing my inner witch in a hugely public way, and these ladies sat with me on a Zoom call without judgement as I let this fear release through (*many*) tears and wails!

Having a cheer squad is invaluable for this type of support, but this does not mean you can shoulder others with the responsibility to take the actions that are yours to take or to manage your emotions for you; for example, only I could release the fear and find the courage to write this book. The ability to self-regulate and be accountable is part of being a woman in her power. Suppressing and struggling in silence is not.

The Witchual

I highly encourage you to build your own cheer squad, focusing especially on including women with whom you feel aligned. The more you connect with these women, the more you will step into your own power, let go of comparison, and trust others.

Your squad could include:

▽ Your family
▽ Your friends
▽ Your colleagues
▽ Your mentor/coach*
▽ Your role models
▽ Your ancestors**
▽ Your spirit guides**

*I recommend only working with one coach or mentor at a time to avoid feeling overwhelmed. Everyone has their own unique approach, so take the time to find someone you really connect with.

**Note: Yes, there are ways to connect with some amazing female figures outside of the physical realm. That will be one of my future books. For now, I highly recommend Sand Symes' *Ancestral Breathwork Journeys* to get started.

With the above in mind, get out your journal or consult the journal pages in the back of this book and make a list of women who you want to enlist in your cheer squad. Then, if you feel called, add any men who you'd also like to join you.

Once you've finished making your list, give it a little audit. Go through each name to make sure your squad only includes those who are going to make you feel fully supported, as opposed to shamed or judged.

Have you considered that others may have different beliefs to you? This doesn't necessarily mean they can't be in your cheer squad; it just may mean they support you differently. My best friend, for example, isn't interested in anything esoteric. And that's totally cool with me! She's still in my squad and supports me in her own way. Remember, it's not your responsibility to persuade others to make moon water with you. It is, however, your choice to invite them to be a part of your journey and be fine with whether they say, "yes" or "no".

How big do you want your cheer squad to be? If you're a very sociable, extroverted person, having 100+ women in your squad probably sounds amazing. If you're like me and are more introverted, it may be preferable to stick to a small, select squad.

You may also find that your initial squad needs some fine-tuning as you progress on your journey, from changing up your reading list as you discover new authors to finding new friends with whom you share an instant deep connection (shout out to my soul sisters Kacie Monroe, Tasha

Trina, and Laura Harding). Keep checking in with yourself. Are you making empowered choices when letting people into your squad?

The Wisdom

Only you can unlock your power and reclaim your inner witch, but this doesn't mean you must do it all on your own. In fact, I'd argue that it's essential that you *don't* do it on your own. Create a cheer squad with amazing women (and men) who you know will support you from the sidelines. I personally love working with clients because of the incredible connection we develop. If you'd like to know more about having me as part of your cheer squad, head to www.reclaimthewitch.com. Be warned: I'm a total witch. But then again, by now, you probably are too.

STEP 8: END THE BATTLE
OF THE *hexes*

The Curse

As you step into your power, it's essential to surround yourself with people with whom you feel aligned. In the last section, I focused on why it's especially important to build authentic, trusting relationships with other women, and this section considers why it's also important to do the same with the men in our lives. I explain why we need to put an end to the concept of "the battle of the sexes" and suggest that men are in fact an important ally as we step into our power.

With the (helpful) rise in awareness of the unique challenges women have historically faced as well as current gender inequalities, there's been a lot of (less helpful) "man bashing." Men are being blamed and shamed for all the terrible things that women have experienced over the centuries —and sometimes continue to experience. As a result, many are feeling attacked and unfairly judged based solely on the fact that they're men.

It goes without saying, but I'm going to say it anyway: most men (like most women) are fundamentally good people. It's not their fault there are a minority of idiot men out there (just as it's not a woman's fault there are some not so nice women in the world), or that generations of men before them were sexist, misogynistic, or afraid to speak up for women's rights.

It's not their responsibility to shoulder the mistakes of others, nor should they be blamed or punished for them simply because they are men. It *is* their responsibility to choose to do things differently. For this to happen, as women, we need to allow them the space to choose to do so and to put down our swords.

We are not at war with men, so let's end this whole "battle of the sexes" thing, for example, when it comes to positive discrimination in the workplace. Of course, fair treatment, equal opportunity, and acknowledgement of our talents are vital regardless of whether we're male or female. However, I cannot get on board with the idea of being hired or paid more purely because I'm a woman.

Despite good intentions, positive discrimination isn't giving men the opportunity to choose to do things differently. They're being forced. No one triumphs in this situation. First off, it's alienating a lot of men who might otherwise be our allies as we step into our feminine power.

It's also breeding the same brand of entitlement that we've been fighting against. The goal is more empowered women, not more entitled women. When we choose empowerment over entitlement, we move beyond the patriarchal system of authority that has for too long given men privileges based solely on their gender. Instead of acting the same as the patriarchy, let's do things differently.

Women are under a lot of pressure because of the current push for positive discrimination, for example, to "break the glass ceiling" in fields where men predominate. However, not all of us want to work in or are energetically aligned with male-dominated fields.

There are some professions that are better suited to people with more masculine energy, and some that are more suited to people with more feminine energy. If I'm losing you a little here, keep reading as I describe the distinction between men and women and masculine and feminine in more detail below.

Naturally, as women, most of us have more feminine energy and therefore thrive in more feminine careers such as nursing, teaching, and coaching. However, some women excel in more traditionally male-dominated professions (like programming and accounting) because they naturally have more masculine energy. The same is true for men; while most have a more masculine energy, some do better in more feminine roles because they have more feminine energy.

I'm not saying women can't or shouldn't be able to make it in a male-dominated industry. What I *am* suggesting is that you get curious about whether this aligns with *your* energy. If so, great. If not, that's okay too. My wish for everyone, men and women, is to feel empowered to make a positive impact in the world in a way that is right for them. I'll go more into how you can achieve this in Step 11: Do What Comes Super-naturally. For now, let's get clear on the distinction between gender (male/female, men/women) and gender-based energies (masculine/feminine).

The Cure

Regardless of our gender, we all have both masculine and feminine energies. Consider them a bit like sound volume dials that you can turn up or down. The degree to which these dials are turned up or down varies for each person. Men tend to have their masculine energy more turned up than women, and women tend to have their feminine energy more turned up than men.

The dials also have distinctive characteristics; they can play diverse types of music. You'll likely see the terms "wounded masculine or feminine" and "divine masculine or feminine" used to represent these. "Wounded masculine or feminine" describes limiting traits, whereas "divine masculine or feminine" describes more expansive traits that help us step into our most powerful, aligned selves. I've listed some examples below.[16]

Wounded masculine	Wounded feminine	Divine masculine	Divine feminine
Controlling	Neediness	Supportive	Intuitive and in
Aggressive	Plays the	Confident	flow
Must win at all	victim	Logical	Authentic
costs	Insecurity	Protects and	Compassionate
Abusive	Manipulative	provides security	Vulnerable
Avoidant	Co-dependent	Honest and	Trusting
Volatile/reactive	Jealous	integral	Creative

With the old patriarchal system, wounded masculine energy has been dialed to the max and the divine feminine completely tuned out, both individually and collectively. Ultimately, this is what we are rebelling against when we talk about feminine empowerment. It's not a matter of a gender battle; it's a matter of dialing up the expansive masculine and feminine energies that reside within us all.

The Witchual

I'm not a man, so I don't know for certain what would help men feel less attacked and judged. If you have any thoughts on this, please share them with me over on Instagram @nutritionbylizzy. I'd love to have this discussion with you and the men in your life who want to genuinely support women in stepping into their power.

Because what I do know is that talking about and becoming clear on the distinction between gender and gender-based energies has been helpful for the men (and women) in my life in understanding where my intention lies as I step into my divine feminine (and masculine) power. If you have similar intentions as me, talking about this topic may also help you and your loved ones.

I encourage you to start engaging the men in your life in conversations around feminine empowerment.

For example, ask:

▽ What does feminine empowerment mean to them?
▽ How does it make them feel?
▽ Would they be open to hearing your perspective?

While it may be tempting to lecture or butt in, just listen and get curious. At the end of the conversation, simply express how grateful you are for them and whatever it is they shared. After all, compassion, gratitude, and curiosity are powerful divine feminine energies!

It's also often the case that what we put out is what we receive back. For example, it's likely you'll find that the more you do this, the more the men you care about and who you want to support you on your journey feel less threatened and more open to discussion around feminine empowerment. They may start asking more about how they can help you or even how they can tap into *their* divine feminine energy.

As a woman stepping into her power, this then gives you the beautiful opportunity to articulate what you need from a place of receptivity and love and model the type of collaborative behavior that will help both you and others step into their power.

It's important to realize that, while we are responsible for communicating our intentions, we are not responsible for other people's reactions, and it's unfair to place expectations regarding how someone *should* react when you talk about this topic.

For example, maybe some men will still feel attacked or threatened by the idea of feminine empowerment. Or maybe they promise to support you from the sidelines but don't want to dive in themselves. That's totally okay. The key is to acknowledge them and be thankful they engaged in the discussion, especially if it's your partner.

Personally, I'm very thankful for my husband; he makes me feel seen, safe, and supported on this journey. My goal is to make love, not war, with him! Are you still battling with the men in your life? Or are you on the same team?

The Wisdom

I'm calling an end to the battle of the sexes right here. Ladies, let's put down our armor and instead work *with* the men in our lives to better understand and support one another. Through engaging men in conversation around feminine empowerment, we can become allies in transmuting wounded masculine energy into expansive masculine and feminine energies. Just imagine what's possible when we collectively do this! However, it all starts with us making the decision to work on ourselves. If you or someone you know (male or female) is ready to do this internal work, head to www.reclaimthewitch.com and book a call with me; I'd love to hear from you.

STEP 9: BE A *Wanderer*

The Curse

In the previous couple of sections, we talked about how having harmonious and aligned relationships is crucial when stepping into your power and reclaiming your inner witch. Your internal environment is directly affected by your external environment, especially if you're someone who is sensitive to their surroundings. I therefore ask you to consider how attuned you are to the people, places and spaces that surround you.

If you're like me, you can quickly get a feel for whether somewhere feels like a good fit for you. The first time I was aware of this was when my mum suggested we visit several universities before I applied to calm my fears about the process (and because wandering around unfamiliar places is fun)!

As the first in my family to apply to university, I expected to feel completely out of place among the academic elite, so I was beyond surprised when we walked around the University of Cambridge. The whole place seemed to have a magical glow to it; the 16th century buildings were as charming and welcoming as the students and professors. I clung to the prospectus all the way home, dreaming about studying there.

The next day, Mum and I battled six hours of traffic, road works, and detours to visit another university, which I thought I'd like even more. The universe was clearly sending me a sign throughout the journey because, as soon as I got out of the car, my stomach dropped, and I realized I hated the place!

"What do you think?" Mum asked, tired but hopeful.

I couldn't lie.

"Okay. At least, let's spend an hour looking around after having made such a trek," she sighed.

Poor Mum!

However, she and I both felt the power of my intuition regarding the places we'd visited. I applied to and was accepted by the University of Cambridge, and I ended up enjoying the university and city so much that I spent eight years studying, working, and living there.

Don't get me wrong, I'm not always great at listening when I have an all-knowing feeling about a place. When I was applying to study for my PhD, I went through the same process of looking at universities as I did when I was applying as an undergraduate. But thanks to the lure of a scholarship and a great academic reputation, my head took over, and I ended up in a place where I felt unbelievably unhappy from the get-go. I tried so hard to make it work, but two apartments, four panic attacks, and six months later, I packed my suitcase and left to move back to Cambridge. As soon as I got off the train and saw the historic buildings, I felt like I'd been reunited with old friends, and my anxiety melted away.

Can you relate? Have you ever had an intuitive feeling about a place, whether that be feeling joyful and comfortable or unhappy and misaligned? Did you listen to and honor that feeling?

Maybe it happened when you were on holiday. Maybe you've found yourself somewhere you didn't expect and loved it. Or maybe you've always wanted to go somewhere but were super disappointed when you finally visited.

As an 18-year-old, I took a spontaneous day trip to Verona while I was staying on the Italian Riviera. I instantly fell in love with this dreamy, romantic city. On the other hand, I'd always wanted to go to San Francisco and jumped at the opportunity to visit during my internship with the UCLA Athletic Department. To my disappointment, I just didn't vibe with the place; even the sourdough was a letdown (and, let me tell you, I *love* sourdough)!

It's often difficult to predict how we're going to feel when we visit somewhere new, so it's natural to have these experiences. Couple this with the fact that everyone's different; how you feel is likely going to differ from how someone else feels in a certain location. You may be reading this and screaming at me right now because you adore San Francisco!

And that's okay. Always listen to and go with what feels good for you as opposed to relying on how you *think* you should feel or what you *think* you should be doing. Remember what I said earlier about our overthinking brain getting in the way?! If you don't feel good in a location, give yourself grace and honor that feeling. This is important because remaining in a place that isn't aligned with you can compromise both your health and your happiness.

When I travelled halfway across the world to be a volunteer at a sea turtle conservation project in Costa Rica, on paper it sounded lovely and very noble of me, but I was doing it because I thought I should. I hadn't considered that I enjoyed my creature comforts and that living in a cement outbuilding without a shower and with barely a roof over my head was *not* my idea of fun.

I still had an eating disorder, so it was difficult for me to eat enough, and the heat was hard on my fragile body. My group wasn't scheduled to leave for another month, but I knew I wasn't up for the task. So, I decided to head home on my own.

It's not the wisest or safest thing to do as a woman in a foreign country where you don't speak the language, so please don't ever do this. However, my experience demonstrates the importance of trusting your intuitive sense; other than helping you out of places that make you miserable, it'll literally help you survive.

As I headed out of the mangroves and back into the city, I was in full survival mode, and my senses, including my intuition, were heightened. This meant that I made good decisions about where I went and who I trusted, which ultimately resulted in my getting home in one piece. The moral of the story; your intuition is powerful, so learn to listen to it.

The Cure

Positioning yourself in places that feel aligned to you contributes to your health, wellbeing, and happiness. And I really can't think of a more important prerequisite to being able to fully step into your power than being healthy, well, and happy.

As you spend time in and interact with your home environment on a regular daily basis, this is perhaps the first and most prominent place to consider when you're assessing whether your surroundings support you in being healthy, well, and happy.

Tony Robbins is famously quoted as saying: "The quality of your life is determined by the quality of questions you ask yourself."[17] Therefore, when it comes to your home environment, start to ask yourself questions such as:

▽ Do you enjoy having a space in your house where you can be outside?

▽ Is it important to you to have a grassy area so that you can take off your shoes and ground yourself?

▽ Do you want to grow flowers and/or herbs?

▽ Do you have the time and energy to maintain a garden?

▽ If you work from home, does your office align with how you want to feel when you show up at work?

▽ Is your desk organized?

▽ Do you have a comfortable office chair to sit on?

▽ Do you have a professional backdrop for your Zoom calls?

▽ Do you value being able to cook yourself nutritious meals, and is your kitchen set up to enable you to do this?

▽ Are your cupboards and fridge stocked with healthy options?

▽ Do you have all the appliances and implements you need to be able to cook your favorite recipes?

Get out your journal and take 10-15 minutes to use these questions to help you assess the type of home environment that feels good for you, whether your current environment is aligned with this, and what needs to change.

The Witchual

The voice of circumstance may jump in to tell you why your current home environment isn't ideal; for example, it may tell me that we live in an apartment in the city of Los Angeles so having the big garden of my dreams isn't possible right now.

Whatever it tells you, the voice of circumstance can feel super disempowering. Don't give your power away; and instead, use your divine feminine power of creativity to explore what *is* possible. For example, I've used our small balcony to create a mini outdoor sanctuary. I grow herbs and potted plants, have hung some wind chimes, and have a couple of nice chairs and a table to sit at as I sip my morning coffee.

Have fun thinking of creative ways to upgrade your home environment so that it's more aligned with how you want to feel. For example, maybe you throw out all the things languishing at the back of your kitchen cupboards that expired two years ago, or maybe you buy a cool new office chair to replace the old, rickety one that hurts your back.

Give this a go for one of the things you identified in your journal as needing to change in your home environment and notice how your energy and behaviors change as a result.

Powerful, isn't it?!

Create an Altar

If you don't already have an alter in your home, I highly recommend creating one as part of this upgrade which you can use for some of your witchuals, and as a daily visual reminder of your power. The beauty of altars is that they can be fully personalized to you and your current circumstance.

I have two altars: one above my desk, which is covered in "thank you" cards from clients, crystals, candles, and my favorite books, with a smudge stick and room spray for energy clearing. Don't worry if you don't know what this is as I'm about to go into more detail on this in a bit.

My other altar is on our balcony, where I keep a notebook, a pen, shells, more crystals, and incense. Other witches I know have created altars in their bedroom, living room, closet, and even in a shoebox if they travel a lot or are short on space. As always, do what works best for you.

The same goes when it comes to deciding what you include on the altar; from photos, cards, and post-it notes to trinkets, wands, and crystals, it's entirely up to you. You can buy items for the altar, but it's not necessary; buying more stuff won't make you a more powerful witch, so don't feel pressured if you're doing this on a budget or don't want to work with certain items.

If you *do* want to buy something- for example, a crystal- shop intuitively. Buy the item that you feel drawn to, not the one that you've been told to get because it has a certain property or meaning. You'll often find that when you look the property or meaning up later, it naturally resonates with you and what you're calling into your life. For example, the crystals I tend to be drawn to are rose quartz (great for self-love), citrine (brings positive, sun-like optimism) and tiger's eye (for luck and prosperity).

Cleanse Your Space

Whenever I perform a ritual at one of my altars, from doing a client call to casting a spell, I like to cleanse the energy of my space so that any residual negativity is removed, and I have more direct access to my powers. My favorite ways to do this are via smudging or using a room spray.

Smudging essentially involves burning a type of sacred herb or resin (the most used are sage and Palo Santo) and wafting the smoke around you and your environment to clear the energies.[18] I like to be a bit extra and prance around the house a little when I do this, but it's totally up to you how you smudge.

Of course, practicing fire safety is important, and if the idea of making smoke in your house makes you nervous, an alternative way to elevate the energy of your space is to use a room spray made of moon water and essential oils. You can download my favorite room spray recipe at www.reclaimthewitch.com.

As with crystals, when it comes to choosing what essential oils to include in your room spray or what herbs to use for smudging, use your intuition to guide you. Yes; it's important to look up the properties of essential oils and herbs on the internet to check if they are safe to use around children and pets. Otherwise, play around, sniff lots of different options, and see what you're drawn to. There's literally no right or wrong here!

There are also no rules on how often or when to use a room spray or smudge to clear the energy of your environment. While I do it whenever I perform a ritual, other witches cleanse their spaces at various times of the year, for example, on equinoxes and solstices; to honor our connection with Mother Earth. I'll be speaking more about this in the next section. Other witches cleanse their space whenever they've had visitors in their house, just in case someone forgets to take their negative energy with them when they leave!

The Wisdom

Our external environment is just as important as our internal environment in helping us to step into our power and embrace our inner witch. Use your home environment to create a surrounding that aligns with your feeling healthy, well, and happy. In this section, I hope I've proved you don't have to wait for circumstance to grant you permission to start. However, if you're still looking for permission to do and create what feels good to you, here's your permission slip. Now, go have fun and head to www.reclaimthewitch.com for my favorite room spray recipe so that you can create your own personal potion for instantly elevating the energy of your home.

STEP 10: *Em-witch* THE EARTH

The Curse

In the previous section, we discussed how important it is to position yourself within an environment that's conducive to you stepping into your power, and I encouraged you to start by considering your home environment. A discussion of our environment, however, feels incomplete if we don't consider beautiful Mother Earth herself. I'll explain in this section why having a connection with her is so crucial for anyone hoping to reclaim their inner witch.

Ever since humans first appeared on this planet, we have relied on the Earth to provide the resources necessary for us to survive—from food to clean water, from fresh air to building materials. Referred to as Mother Nature, Mother Earth, or Pachamama in some indigenous cultures, the Earth is like a mother to us all, creating and sustaining life.[19] She is abundant, fertile, and loves us deeply.

However, her love hasn't always been reciprocated by us humans, particularly in the last few centuries. Industrialization, population growth, and greed have meant that, as a species, we've taken increasingly from the Earth.

In doing so, we've raped her of resources, shrunk her natural habitats, and forced her to produce year-round, non-stop. We've poisoned her water and air, pushed other species to extinction, and dysregulated the delicate balance in the climate that we so often take for granted.

The statistics speak for themselves. Since the beginning of the 20th century, birds, mammals, and amphibians have been going extinct 100 to 1000 times faster than average. Alarmingly, many scientists think this could be an underestimation because many species are understudied, and their numbers are difficult to predict.[20]

Meanwhile, from 1750 to 2020, the average global carbon dioxide concentration increased by 49%[21] and, in that same period, the world lost a total of 1.5 billion hectares of forest. For those who think visually like me, that's one and a half times the size of the United States.[22] Our impact on the Earth over the last 300 years has been so profound that scientists suggest we are in a new geological period: the Anthropocene (anthro meaning "human").[23]

As I write this, I can't help but notice the parallels between how, as a collective, we've been (mis)treating Mother Earth and how we've been (mis)treating our feminine energy. Both are attempts to exert dominance over, subdue, and restrain the nourishing, creative life force that surrounds and resides within us all. If we continue the same narrative, we risk messing things up for ourselves as well as future generations.

You only need to look back over the past 300 years (and beyond) to see how the simultaneous destruction of Earth and the suppression of feminine energy affected past generations. Our ancestors developed mental and physical illnesses, became disconnected from the environment and each other, and forgot about the incredible magic we have the power to weave in tandem with Mother Earth.

It's time to change this for ourselves *and* our children, don't you agree?

The Cure

I don't tend to get on my soapbox often, but these issues are as close to my heart as they are intertwined. My goal here is not to preach but to share my passions for the Earth and feminine energy and, in turn, help ignite a similar spark in you so that you can rekindle your relationship with them both and fully step into your power.

From gardening with my grandad as a kid to studying natural sciences at university to going on trips to the mountains with my husband, I have always *loved* being in and learning about nature. This sense of wonder and joy is essential if we want to reconnect with the earth, be in tune with our environment, and, as a result, reclaim the witch within.

I encourage you to take a moment to consider: What about the natural world do *you* love? Get out your journal and make a list.

Maybe you love something as simple as the sound of birds singing in the morning or the light tapping of rain on your windowpanes at night. Maybe you get so much joy from putting your hands in the soil and planting seeds, herbs, and flowers. Maybe your shoulders drop a little when you walk on the beach or in a forest. Whatever it is, let your inner witch be in total admiration of all the earth magic that surrounds her.

The seasons particularly fascinate me. I like to think of them as having distinct personalities. Winter is cold, dark, and introspective. Spring has a sense of optimism and freshness, while summer is bold and full-on. Autumn is my favorite, with its changeability and colorful nature. Getting to know these different personalities has been a game changer in unlocking my power.

That's because, as we now know, just like the seasons, women are naturally cyclic. In fact, we can think of womanhood and the changes we experience in our bodies over our lifetimes as being divided into four distinct phases that reflect the four seasons.

Our formative years are like spring; it's a time of naïve enthusiasm and huge growth. When we become adults, we transition into the summer of life; we are fertile and exude a magnetic, irresistible energy. When we reach mid-life, we can experience huge changes (for example, children leave home and we go through menopause), just as in autumn. And then finally, in the winter of our lives, we are raw, unapologetic, and embrace death as a natural part of life.

Season	Life stage*	Menstrual phase	Personality
Spring	Childhood and Teens	Pre-ovulation	Energetic, enthusiastic, outgoing
Summer	Adulthood	Ovulation	Bold, magnetic, fertile
Autumn	Mid-life	Pre-menstruation	Wise, temperamental, honest
Winter	Elder	Menstruation	Inward, reflective, unapologetic

*Elsewhere, you may see these referred to as Maiden, Mother, Wild Woman, and Crone. However, I've chosen what I consider more empowering and inclusive terms to describe the four main life stages women go through.

I've illustrated how the seasons correspond to our different life stages in the table above. I've also included a column indicating how the seasons, just like the phases of the moon, reflect each stage of our menstrual cycle. Our bodies mirror the seasons in many ways. Understanding this is not only poetic but also super powerful because it creates an opportunity for us to give ourselves a little grace and compassion, which we so often neglect to do.

It also means we can tap into our strengths as we cycle physically, energetically, emotionally, and physiologically from month to month and year to year. For example, during my inner spring and summer, I know I'm going to have more energy and drive to be out in the world. I plan more social engagements for this time and honor my enjoyment of more intense activities like running.

In contrast, during my inner autumn and winter, I tend to get cozy, politely decline social invitations, and retreat inward to do more restful activities such as yoga and being creative. This allows me to recharge and come back to the beginning of my cycle, my inner spring, nurtured and ready to bloom.

The Witchual

Reconnecting with the cycles and the seasons within and around you are vital for reclaiming your inner witch. However, this process is so beautifully personal and unique to you. For example, our personal season may not always correspond to our current life stage or Mother Earth's current season. And, while one woman is going through her winter, another woman will be going through her spring.

As I've also mentioned many, many times in this book, there are no rules when it comes to stepping into your power. It's about learning what feels good for you and trusting yourself enough to do that. So, while I invite you to use some of my favorite ways to reconnect with and intertwine with the wisdom of Mother Earth and her seasonal cycles, I also encourage you to get creative and come up with some of your own rituals.

I find rituals that bring my physical body into contact with Mother Earth are the most potent for helping me recharge my magic. For example, I love going on regular nature walks and finding a place where I can put my bare feet in the grass for 5 to 10 minutes (a practice known as grounding). When I can't find a patch of grass (because, let's face it, I live in Los Angeles, so it can be tricky), I do the same thing at the beach.

Meanwhile, I plant herbs on our balcony, which I harvest and use in my homemade remedies. Some clients come to me because they're experiencing digestive issues such as gas, constipation, acid reflux, and IBS. Fermented food and drink products like kombucha are an excellent natural way to give our guts a boost because of the probiotics they contain.[24] While you can buy kombucha from the store, it's way more fun to make your own and play around with making different flavor combinations using homegrown ingredients (my favorite combo is lemon and thyme).

I also honor the seasons by observing the Wheel of the Year. The Wheel of the Year marks the prominent astrological placements of the earth relative to the sun and is centered around the summer and winter solstices, as well as the spring and autumn equinoxes. Halfway between the solstices and the equinoxes are the entry points to each season, also known as cross-quarter days or fire gateways. These are Imbolc, Beltane, Lammas, and Samhain.

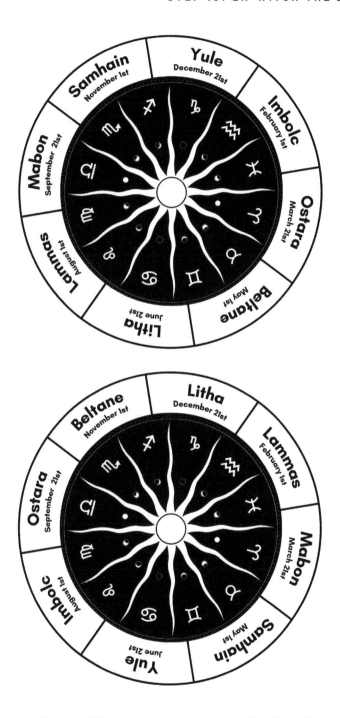

Top image: Northern Hemisphere, Bottom image: Southern Hemisphere

While the dates vary slightly from year to year (so be sure to double check), the table below gives you an idea of when to mark your calendars so that you can celebrate each point on the Wheel of the Year. Of course, you can do this in whatever way you choose.

	Northern Hemisphere	Southern Hemisphere
Winter Solstice ('Yule')	December 21st	June 21st
Imbolc	February 1st	August 1st
Spring Equinox ('Ostara')	March 21st	September 21st
Beltane	May 1st	November 1st
Summer Solstice ('Litha')	June 21st	December 21st
Lammas	August 1st	February 1st
Autumn Equinox ('Mabon')	September 21st	March 21st
Samhain	November 1st	May 1st

Observing the Wheel of the Year is a wonderful opportunity to celebrate the flora, fauna, and energies unique to that point in the earth's annual cycle around the sun. For example, at the autumn equinox, I celebrate the harvest. This is a time when I pick apples from the local orchards and turn them into sauces and baked oatmeal, all while giving thanks to Mother Nature for keeping us fed.

Acknowledging these eight points during the year is an easy and fun way to stay connected to, celebrate, and work in sync with Mother Earth's cycles. There is already so much written about how to celebrate each of the eight points on the Wheel of the Year; my Instagram feed used to be full of ideas. This got to the point of being overwhelming, so I've decided not to regurgitate this information here and instead want to encourage you to explore the festivals of the land where you currently live and craft your own rituals.

The Wisdom

Being able to recognize and connect with the unique cycles within and surrounding you unlocks a pathway to understanding and trusting yourself, your body, and your magic. It allows you to turn your back on the masculine, linear model of how we "should" function and instead find a way that works for you and your natural rhythms.

It also creates space for play and exploration; for example, I love experimenting with my homemade kombucha. If you're looking for an easy and fun way to boost your gut health so that you can feel good in mind and body, head to www.reclaimthewitch.com and claim my personal kombucha recipe.

By creating more play and finding alignment with your natural rhythms, you'll feel less burnt out and stressed and more energized, relaxed, and at home within yourself. As a result, your authentic feminine power can flourish. Not only will this benefit your health, wellness, and career, but also your relationships with others, including Mother Earth herself.

STEP 11: DO WHAT COMES

super-naturally

The Curse

Self-trust has been a key theme throughout this book because it's the ultimate ingredient to living a magical and empowered life. But I get it; it can be difficult, and despite reading this far, you may still be questioning your innate wisdom. Learning to trust my own inner GPS was one of my most challenging life lessons, and being completely honest, I still don't always listen to it!

Like a petulant child, I can get stuck asking, "Why? Why? Why?" while the universe sits there like a patient parent as if to say, "It's ok; you'll understand when you're older." Can you relate? Like any parent, though, there will come a time when the universe snaps back at you for always questioning and not trusting yourself. When that happens, you had better watch out! The universe *will* intervene. It probably won't feel good, but it'll be what you need.

This is exactly how I came to write this book. Soon after releasing *Reclaim the Rebel*, I had an all-knowing feeling that I would write another book.

The pure bliss I felt from knowing I was helping people with my words reverberated deep within my soul. But my head told me that I needed to wait, and instead of writing, I put all my energy and finances into learning how to grow my business.

It was an uphill battle. I lost a lot of money chasing something that I wasn't truly guided to do. I also wasted a ton of time, mental energy, and stress trying to figure out why all the lead magnets, courses, and podcasts I was creating weren't getting me anywhere, when the answer was simple: I wasn't doing what was aligned with me. This meant that no matter how hard I worked, I was not going to make *it* work.

The longer I resisted, the longer I suffered, and the more the universe screamed at me with signs to trust myself. I wasn't attracting more clients, and one person came close to swindling me out of $9000 by pretending to be a client a week before my wedding. It hurt so badly and felt incredibly scary, but being the stubborn, headstrong witch I am, I kept going.

Then, the opportunity for me to invest in a coaching program came along. I had a deep inner knowing that I was going to be fine without it. However, my head got in the way. I got FOMO and worried that I didn't have all the tools I needed to successfully grow my business. I convinced myself that this program *must* have the answer.

Not only was this a huge disservice to my intuition, but it was also unfair to put that expectation on the program provider. Just a few weeks after investing in it, I realized I really did not need the course, just like my intuition had told me from the start. What a costly but important lesson *that* was.

Things had finally gotten to the point where the pain of my situation outweighed the pain of change; I was broken, had no clients, and was super resentful of the $3600 investment I'd just made. It was a blessing in disguise because these "dark nights of the soul" are when transformation happens—for me, for my clients, for us all. Can you think of a time in your life when the pain of a situation became so great that you had no choice but to do something different?

If so, you'll know that when you get to this tipping point, it's not an easy time. You may feel a deluge of emotions, including fear, anger, disappointment, desperation, resignation, and more fear. If you're like me, you'll probably feel like you're being broken open. Let it happen. In opening, you're creating space to release what no longer serves you. Even if it feels messy and there are tears and snot and ugly crying, let it happen.

Most importantly, be kind to yourself. This is not the time to get judgy and come down hard about how you 'should' have known better or done things differently. No, this is all happening for you, and there's a lesson to be learned. Get curious about what that lesson is. In my case, the lesson was to get out of my own way and use my superpower, writing, as opposed to trying to do what I felt I *should* be doing.

We can get so caught up in the "*should,*" can't we? In *Reclaim the Rebel*, I talk about how this is a result of comparing ourselves to others. But what we often forget is that we are all unique, from our appearance to our abilities, and so this comparison game is futile. In fact, when it comes to our abilities, our superpowers often lie in our unique life challenges.

English literature was my weakest subject in high school (the perfectionist in me was horrified that I only got an A as opposed to an A+ like in all my other subjects) and reading always felt like a chore; as a kid, I never managed to finish a book. This made me feel stupid, lazy, and embarrassed whenever I had to read a book for class.

I also held my pen differently than everyone else. In elementary school, my teachers tried to use all sorts of methods to make me write normally. My stubbornness won and thank goodness it did. I just hate the thought of a little girl being stripped of her uniqueness, don't you?

However, my self-esteem took a real beating in the process. In addition to coming in last on spelling tests (and having to report this publicly in front of my peers), one time a teacher pulled me to the front of the room because I was mispronouncing my "f." She told me to stand there, practicing until I got it right, with 32 pairs of eyes staring at me. I was only seven years old.

No one got curious about my idiosyncrasies. They just wanted to stamp them out. It wasn't until I was preparing to study for my master's in nutrition at King's College London that someone started to ask better questions. During a meeting with the postgraduate disability coordinator about my extreme anxiety, she brought up the possibility that I might be dyslexic.

Apparently, it's common for individuals who have generalized anxiety disorder to also be dyslexic. I like learning, especially about myself (as you're discovering, it's a super powerful thing to do), so I agreed to go for a dyslexia assessment.

Those three hours were *the* most uncomfortable in the whole of my education. At that point, I'd banked stunning grades from school and as an undergraduate at university. I'd also recently qualified as a teacher and been studying for a PhD. But this dyslexia test made me feel like I barely knew the alphabet.

At the end, I hesitantly looked over to the super nice lady administering the assessment and noticed her jaw was halfway down to the floor. And not in the judgmental "you're so dumb" way I was expecting.

"How have you managed to get this far in your academic studies without anyone identifying you as dyslexic?" she gasped.

In that moment, I felt so validated.

"Oh," I thought. "I guess I'm *not* stupid after all."

Finally, I knew why I struggled with reading and writing. It wasn't about the diagnosis; it was about knowing myself that little bit more and being able to use this to my advantage. Understanding I was dyslexic created space for more self-compassion and encouraged me to find ways I could support myself (and the university could support me) in my studies.

I didn't let my dyslexia define me or use the diagnosis to wallow in victimhood or as an excuse not to read or write. In fact, I began to love reading and writing because I gave myself permission to take my time and do things a little differently than other people. The more I relaxed into what felt natural to me, the better I became, especially at writing, and the more I revealed my superpower.

The Cure

The journey of surrendering to what feels natural isn't always easy. It requires you to have an intimate understanding of yourself and the courage of conviction to let go if something feels misaligned and make room for the things that *do* feel good.

As with everything else I've discussed in this book, having self-awareness and taking aligned action are essential for unlocking your power. Get skilled at being aware of when you're feeling out of alignment, asking yourself what action you could take to move you back into what does feel good, taking that action quickly and decisively, and trusting that things will work out (they always do). You'll save yourself a lot of time, money, and energy this way.

You don't need to ask "why?" or "how?" Don't get me wrong; it's good to be curious. It's the doubting and overthinking that will tie you up in knots and result in the exact opposite of action: paralysis. It all comes back to trusting the intuitive nudges, following the path that feels best in that moment, and letting everything come naturally without forcing it or having to know an exact five-point plan for how to get to your destination.

Learning this takes a lifetime of work, not necessarily because it's hard, but because you are human. Things *will* come up that will test whether you can trust yourself to take that aligned action. The trick is to find tools so that you can move through these times with more ease. It's a practice, and with any practice, you will get more confident and competent the more you do it.

Ultimately, only you know when you feel out of alignment. Maybe you feel it in your body, maybe you notice your mood has shifted, or maybe it's something entirely else. Personally, I become super reactive, my body goes into fight or flight mode, and my motivation to engage with whatever or whoever is misaligned with me plummets. Maybe you can relate, or maybe not. Only you know how being out of alignment feels for you.

You're also the only one who knows what would get you back on track, and it's your responsibility to take that action to realign yourself. As much as I love to help, I cannot do this part for you.

However, I *can* give you tools to help you know who you are, unlock your natural powers, and step into your purpose (also known as your dharma). Think of these tools as your North Star, guiding you throughout your life's journey. Whenever you start to feel off track (because, hey, it happens), these tools can put you back on course.

The Witchual

Astrology

So many of us are drawn to horoscopes because they promise to tell us about who we are and how our lives are going to play out. However, mainstream horoscopes like the ones you see in magazines and on social media suffer from the same issue we've been talking about throughout this book: the one-size-fits-all approach. For that reason, you may be skeptical of astrology and how it can help you as an individual.

This is where it's especially useful to know your natal chart (the exact position of the sun, moon, and planets and the astrological aspects when you were born). Your natal chart is completely unique to you and is based on the date, time, and location of where you were born.[25] While your natal chart is literally the map of the sky at the time and place of your birth, you can also think of it as your unique pawn in the game of life. With the help of an expert, you can decipher what natural strengths (and weaknesses) this unique pawn gives you due to the specific placements and aspects in your chart.

Having your natal chart read to you doesn't necessarily tell you anything new, but it does give you extra permission (if you're still looking for it) to fully step into what feels aligned with you. For example, after my reading, I started to fully embrace my need for being among the trees and my play-in-the-dirt Earthiness (my sun is in Taurus). I realized how important it is to tell my story so that I can help others on their health and wellness journeys (Gemini, second house; Virgo, sixth house; Aquarius, eleventh house). I reignited my love of being creative and utilizing it as a way of expressing myself (Leo fifth house), and I accepted that I needed intimate, deep connections in my relationships (Scorpio seventh house).

I'm not an expert in astrology but learning about it and using it as a tool to learn about myself has been super fun and fascinating. It's also been useful to see how my natal chart plays out against current celestial events. If your natal chart is the piece that you play with in the game of life, the transits are what this piece interacts with as you play out that game. Knowing how this interaction is being played out is another element of getting to know yourself at a deep level and fostering more self-awareness, self-compassion, and self-trust.

If you're new to astrology, I highly recommend starting by reaching out to my friend and expert astrologer, Rini York, to get your natal chart read.[26] She's phenomenal at what she does, and I trust she will be able to support you on your spiritual journey as she has with me and countless others.

Human Design

Unlike astrology, when I was first introduced to human design, I wasn't a fan. Human design combines astrology, the I Ching, Kabbalah, and Vedic philosophy and is centered around the idea that there are five energy types (projector, generator, manifestor, reflector, and manifesting generator). These represent five diverse ways humans have been designed to exchange energy with their environment.[27]

I didn't like human design because I discovered I'm a "projector," somebody who does well to rest and wait for someone else to invite them to share their wisdom and expertise. As a former over-doer, I was furious about being categorized as someone who does well doing the exact opposite of what I had predominantly been doing!

However, the more I reflected on how my life has panned out, the more I realized that when I looked after myself, just showed up and did what I loved, and let the people I'm meant to help come to me, I thrived. On the other hand, when I chased the invitation, worked as hard as I could, and put in all the effort, I didn't succeed, I felt bitter, and I burned out.

Apparently, this is common for projectors who are conditioned to operate like generators. Generators are another energy type and work completely differently from projectors (my husband is a generator); they can go for longer periods without rest and are able to create things more consistently. Jealous much? Okay, maybe I am a little.

When I realized and truly embraced the fact that each individual functions differently, I could stop being so hard on myself, step into my power, and use my strengths to my advantage. For example, I need more breaks during my workday than my husband, but when I *am* working, I'm more efficient. Again, it wasn't necessarily that human design has taught me something new about myself, but it has given me the space and permission to do what works best for me.

Just as I'm not an expert in astrology, I'm also not an expert in human design, so I'm not going to try to teach it to you or read your unique chart. Instead, I recommend you book a session with the amazing Barbara Ditlow[28] who trained under the creator of human design, Ra Uru Hu. Within five minutes of talking with her, I gained so much insight into myself. I know that when you talk with her, you will too.

The Heroine's Journey

Do you like watching movies? Me too!

Despite my eclectic taste (my favorites range from *Legally Blonde* to *The Matrix*), most movies follow an archetypal story pattern. You may have noticed it. The main character sets off on their journey, where they encounter a series of challenges. Eventually, they find a way of overcoming these challenges. They then share what they have learned along the way so that others can benefit from their experience. This is what Joseph Campbell called the "Hero's Journey"[29] and, for us witches, I call the "Heroine's Journey."

The "Heroine's Journey" doesn't just apply to Hollywood films. No, sis. It's also the pattern your life has taken (often multiple times).

I'll use an example from my own life. As a teenager, naivety, bullying, and bad advice from magazines resulted in an eating disorder that lasted a decade. Along my journey, I encountered a series of tools that helped me reclaim unconditional love for my body. In *Reclaim the Rebel*, I share these tools so that you can silence your inner mean girl, stop dieting, and feel good in your body even if you've been at war with it for years.

Identifying your "Heroine's Journey" can be a fantastic way to get clear on who you are and what your purpose in life is. Grab your journal to reflect on the following questions:

▽ If your life were a movie, what would the storyline be?

▽ Where did you struggle in the past?

▽ What did you discover during this struggle?

▽ What do you have to share that would benefit other people who are currently going through similar struggles?

What I love most about the "Heroine's Journey" is that it reflects the fact that our superpowers are revealed to us naturally over time, and that we're in a constant state of evolution and transformation. Nothing about the process is forced, and there are no right or wrong routes to discovery. It might get messy and complicated, but that's the beauty of surrendering to our unique life experiences.

Flow State

Surrendering helps things come naturally to us. In fact, this can create moments of extreme clarity and focus, and cause time to get stretchy. This is called being in a "flow state" and is most commonly discussed in relation to professional athletes.[30]

We can all, however, achieve flow states in a variety of ways. For example, I can sit and write for what seems like minutes when in fact it's been hours. Words and ideas cascade through me and onto the page, and as soon as I walk away from my desk, another idea starts to come in. Everything feels so easy and enjoyable when I'm in my flow state. It's even more delicious than a slab of 70% chocolate. Yes, *really*!

What flows super-naturally through you?

Don't force anything if you don't know how to enter a flow state. Simply identify the pursuits that cause you to lose track of time and make time in your schedule to engage in them. Then, watch the magic unfold!

The Wisdom

When we allow our lives to naturally play out, we discover our superpowers and can use them for good in the world. I hope that by sharing some of my experience and the resources that have been beneficial to me throughout this book, you will feel equipped to unlock your own power and rediscover your inner witch. If so, I'd love to hear from you. DM me @nutritionbylizzy on Instagram and share your experiences and key takeaways with me.

EVERY LITTLE THING

SHE DOES IS *magic*

You are magic, sister.

This book wasn't written to tell you how to be magical, because you already are. Just like Little Lizzy, who shared that she was a witch on the playground, deep down, at your core, you know this.

The problem is that over the years, you've forgotten your power and instead have been made to feel "not good enough" or ashamed of who you are. This illusion means that big companies can make money from you, and the patriarchy can keep you in line.

Time to change that and embrace your magic, don't you agree?

If you're ever in doubt that you are already powerful, just think about the all-time classic movie, *The Wizard of Oz*. The characters all felt they lacked something, and so they went on a mission to seek the "guru," the Wizard, to fix this. The Wizard gave each character a tool to help them *feel* whole, but it turns out they were whole all along.

I'm not a guru. I'm just a fellow witch on the same path as you with tools to share that will help you recognize and release your inner power so that you can stop looking for outside validation, start believing in your own inner wisdom, and reclaim unconditional love for your body without wasting any more time, money, or effort on products and personal development courses.

Some of these tools, like those that concern your nutrition, movement, spells, and dreams, can transform the relationship you have with yourself and support your internal environment. Meanwhile, external support, such as friends and partnerships, the places and spaces in which you situate yourself, and Mother Earth and her seasons, can help you live in alignment with your innate magic and feel safe to express it.

You don't have to agree with everything I say or implement all the suggestions I share in this book. In fact, I kind of hope you don't. Because the beauty of a woman in her power is that she is entirely unique, and she gets to decide what's best for her. So, while it's an honor to guide you on your journey of rediscovering your magic, unlocking your power, and loving your body, ultimately, it's *your* journey, and it will probably look different from mine.

I highly recommend creating a daily routine that's personalized to you; for example, journaling your dreams and tracking your menstrual cycle; spending 10 to 15 minutes doing self-hypnosis; and regularly tuning into your body's subtle signals when it comes to choosing how you move and nourish it.

The most important message I want you to take away from this book is to take actions that feel good and empower you and your body. In doing this, give yourself permission to mess up and to succeed in equal measure.

Now, go work that wand and make some magic!

THE *witch* IS BACK

Hi, I'm Lizzy Cangro!

I'm a multi-award-winning author, expert nutritionist, and wellness witch whose passion and purpose are to help women access and embrace the power and magic housed within their incredible female bodies.

Holding an MA in Natural Sciences from the University of Cambridge and an MSc in Nutrition from King's College London, I combine science with an empathetic understanding and a side of "woo woo" wisdom to help you let go of the anxiety of not feeling "enough" and confidently step into the body you love.

My goal is to help as many women as possible achieve more inner peace, joy, and love for themselves. In doing so, I want to contribute to the growing movement whereby women can unite and let go of the shame and distrust we have towards our bodies and each other.

Will you join me?

Learn more about how to work with me and download your complimentary Reclaim the Witch resources at www.reclaimthewitch.com.

Witch NOTES

ACKNOWLEDGEMENTS

Thank you to my husband, Steve, for supporting me as I step into my power. I can't fully put into words how much I appreciate everything you do. Thank you also to my editor, Traci Hohenstein, for so lovingly supporting me through the creation of this book.

ENDNOTES

1 https://www.countrylife.co.uk/nature/history-elder-tree-deities-dryads-shakespeare-j-k-rowling-197720

2 https://www.space.com/beaver-moon-lunar-eclipse-photos-november-2021

3 https://www.linkedin.com/pulse/95-5-rule-michele-molitor-cpcc-pcc-rtt-c-hyp/?trk=portfolio_article-card_title

4 https://www.thespruce.com/black-onyx-used-in-feng-shui-1274362

5 https://ishka.com/blogs/spirit/tree-of-life-symbolism

6 https://kidshealth.org/en/kids/menstruation.html

7 https://www.womenshealth.gov/menopause/menopause-basics

8 https://www.livescience.com/intermittent-fasting-for-women

9 https://www.kidcentraltn.com/development/8-10-years/brain-development-ages-8-10.html)

10 https://www.ncdhhs.gov/about/department-initiatives/early-childhood/why-early-childhood-matters)

11 https://www.scientificamerican.com/article/fact-or-fiction-lead-can-be-turned-into-gold/

12 https://www.newsweek.com/adele-reveals-backlash-weight-loss-says-some-fans-felt-betrayed-1721442)

13 https://www.theguardian.com/commentisfree/2022/nov/01/was-taylor-swift-wrong-to-use-the-word-fat-in-a-video-thats-how-i-used-to-feel-whenever-i-weighed-myself

14 https://www.history.com/topics/folklore/history-of-witches

15 https://www.washingtonpost.com/national/health-science/study-finds-that-fear-can-travel-quickly-through-generations-of-mice-dna/2013/12/07/94dc97f2-5e8e-11e3-bc56-c6ca94801fac_story.html

16 https://sarahalnoon.com/blog-posts/healing-balancing-masculine-feminine-within-us-energies-divine-wounded

17 Anthony Robbins, *Awaken the Giant Within*

18 https://www.thespruce.com/how-to-smudge-your-house-1274692

19 https://en.wikipedia.org/wiki/Pachamama

20 https://ourworldindata.org/extinctions

21 https://www.co2.earth/global-co2-emissions)

22 https://ourworldindata.org/habitat-loss

23 https://ourworldindata.org/extinctions

24 https://www.brewdrkombucha.com/blog/kombucha-vs-probiotic-supplements-which-is-best/

25 https://en.wikipedia.org/wiki/Horoscope

26 https://divine.riniheart.com

27 https://en.wikipedia.org/wiki/Human_Design

28 https://humandesignconsultations.com/schedule/

29 https://en.wikipedia.org/wiki/Hero%27s_journey

30 https://www.verywellmind.com/what-is-flow-2794768

CPSIA information can be obtained
at www.ICGtesting.com
Printed in the USA
JSHW080829300523
42311JS00002B/100